Pharmaceutical Care Issues of Patients with Rheumatoid Arthritis

Louise Grech • Alan Lau
Editors

Pharmaceutical Care Issues of Patients with Rheumatoid Arthritis

From Hospital to Community

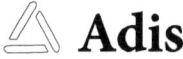 Adis

Editors
Louise Grech
Department of Pharmacy
University of Malta
Msida
Malta

Alan Lau
Pharmacy Practice
International Clinical Pharmacy Education
University of Illinois at Chicago
Chicago
Illinois
USA

ISBN 978-981-10-1420-8   ISBN 978-981-10-1421-5   (eBook)
DOI 10.1007/978-981-10-1421-5

Library of Congress Control Number: 2016944493

Printed on acid-free paper

This Adis imprint is published by Springer Nature
The registered company is Springer Science+Business Media Singapore Pte Ltd.

Dedicated to all rheumatoid arthritis patients

Foreword

Management of patients with rheumatoid arthritis (RA) is often carried out subjectively by healthcare professionals, sometimes, resulting in less than optimal outcomes. This book undertakes to shift practice from these systems towards meeting patients' needs whilst responding to economic, regulatory and pharmaceutical care forces, using clinical experience while following the rules of evidence.

The goals of this book are to enhance pharmacists' ability to make intelligent professional judgements regarding best practices in RA with emphasis on the patient, drawing on the knowledge of drug therapy, and to encourage the development of specialisation within pharmacy practice in RA without neglecting the holistic approach to patient care. These goals are achieved by giving examples of ways to extend the pharmacists' practice from hospitals to other settings through seamless care. All these functions may be reached through the stimulation of two pillars of academia, namely, teaching and research activities and their relevance to translational medicine as regards the evolving specialisation of RA.

The outcomes expected from reading and actually following the contents of this book include: (1) to make pharmacists more sophisticated in their knowledge of RA, (2) to enhance the ability to put forward intelligent judgements regarding pharmacotherapeutic pathways for each individual patient, based on patient characteristics, while taking into consideration pharmacoeconomic and distribution systems within a national health service, (3) to stimulate pharmacists both in hospital and community settings to incorporate pharmaceutical care algorithms in the broad concept of patient care, (4) to promote systematic, albeit, flexible innovate ways to approach RA therapy through the introduction of evidence-based tools such as the RhMAT, Rheumatoid Arthritis Medication Assessment Tool, approach as part of the pharmaceutical care model, (5) to spearhead new patterns of clinical pharmacy practice with emphasis on teamwork approach by using RA as a model, (6) to bring significant historical and social points to the attention of professionals such as highlighting the misconception of confusing arthritis with RA, and (7) to encourage students, clinicians and academia to review teaching and research activities in the area of RA. These outcomes may be achieved by following the particular characteristics of this book, which are often stand-alone reads and self-explanatory. These caveats include a description of clinical manifestations, a table on laboratory investigations, classification criteria based on ACR-EULAR guidelines, early diagnosis and pyramid pharmacological treatment systems, essential features of drugs available with dosage regimens, contraindications and side effects, and a summary of treatment strategies. Since the application of pharmacoeconomic principles plays a pivotal role in the treatment of RA, especially with the development of biologicals and new cost-saving biosimilars, a whole chapter dedicated to pharmacoeconomics is well in order. This chapter carries a number of case studies, some of them were met by the authors in their practice as are other case studies throughout the text.

Finally, a significant contribution of this book to the management of RA is the highlighting of how pharmaceutical care issues particularly the description of how the RhMAT, as an innovative tool, can be incorporated to support patient seamless care. In particular, the take-home messages found throughout the chapters provide features that should be considered to be adopted in day-to-day practice.

Msida, Malta   Anthony Serracino-Inglott

Preface

There are various textbooks and literature available on rheumatoid arthritis and its pharmacotherapy. This book, edited by Louise Grech and Alan Lau, two pharmacists with a strong background of clinical pharmacy and pharmaceutical care incorporates the theoretical aspects of rheumatoid arthritis into the real-life scenario focusing on the clinical and pharmaceutical care aspects of rheumatoid arthritis patients.

This book is mainly aimed at pharmacy students but can also be used as a reference by other healthcare professionals in contact with rheumatoid arthritis patients. It is a comprehensive guide introducing the readers to the very basic aspects of rheumatoid arthritis, helping them understand its clinical significance and impact of this disease on the patients' activities of daily living. The clinical practical scenarios presented enable the readers to easily follow the text and allows the introduction of the concept of pharmaceutical care of rheumatoid arthritis extending to the community care setting. What is salutary is that it helps students to come to terms with the practical aspect of managing and caring for a rheumatoid arthritis patient.

This book also places an emphasis on communication which is required by all the healthcare professionals who need to work together and with rheumatoid arthritis patients. This joint collaboration between authors from different settings emphasises the concept of joint care between clinicians and pharmacists, as this is surely the way to providing patients with the best quality of care service.

Msida, Malta   Godfrey LaFerla

Acknowledgements

First and foremost I would like to thank the contributors of this publication, without whom this book would not have been possible. I would also like to acknowledge the support received from my colleagues, at the Clinical Pharmacy Practice Unit at Mater Dei Hospital, in particular the medicines information pharmacists. My gratitude is also due to all the staff and colleagues at the Department of Pharmacy and the Faculty of Medicine and Surgery at the University of Malta. A special thank you goes to the patients who agreed to share their experiences giving this book a real-life scenario twist. On a personal note, I would like to thank my family and close friends for supporting me in each venture. A massive thank you to the publishers of this book who gave us this challenging opportunity to come together as coauthors and present this book to capture the essentials of pharmaceutical care aspects of rheumatoid arthritis to readers. Finally I would like to deeply thank Professor Alan Lau, University of Illinois, Chicago, for his invaluable contribution as my coeditor.

Msida, Malta   Louise Grech

Contents

1   **Understanding Rheumatoid Arthritis**.   1
     Carmel Mallia and Bernard Coleiro

2   **Pharmacotherapy of Rheumatoid Arthritis**. 19
     Aygin Bayraktar-Ekincioglu and Louise Grech

3   **Pharmacoeconomics and Rheumatoid Arthritis** 39
     Maurice Zarb Adami and Bernard Coleiro

4   **Pharmaceutical Care Issues of Rheumatoid Arthritis Patients** 53
     Lilian M. Azzopardi, Louise Grech, and Marilyn Rogers

5   **Transitional Care: Caring Across the Interface**. 71
     Karen Farrugia and Margarida Caramona

**Conclusion: Teaching Pharmaceutical Care of Rheumatoid
Arthritis Patients to Student Practitioners: Imparting Care** 79

Glossary 83

Index 85

Contributors

Maurice Zarb Adami, PhD Department of Pharmacy, Faculty of Medicine and Surgery, University of Malta, Msida, Malta

Lilian M. Azzopardi, PhD Department of Pharmacy, Faculty of Medicine and Surgery, European Association of Faculties of Pharmacies, University of Malta, Msida, Malta

Aygin Bayraktar-Ekincioglu, PhD Department of Clinical Pharmacy, Faculty of Pharmacy, Hacettepe University, Ankara, Turkey

Margarida Caramona, PhD Faculty of Pharmacy, European Association of Faculties of Pharmacies, University of Coimbra, Coimbra, Portugal

Bernard Coleiro, MD, FRCP, M.Phil (Melit) Faculty of Medicine and Surgery, University of Malta, Msida, Malta

Department of Medicine, Mater Dei Hospital, Msida, Malta

Karen Farrugia, BPharm (Hons) (Melit) Chemimart Group of Pharmacies, Msida, Malta

Louise Grech, PhD Clinical Pharmacy Practice Unit, Department of Pharmacy, Mater Dei Hospital, Msida, Malta

Department of Pharmacy, Faculty of Medicine and Surgery, University of Malta, Msida, Malta

Alan Lau, PharmD, FCCP Pharmacy Practice, International Clinical Pharmacy Education, University of Illinois, Chicago (UIC) College of Pharmacy, Chicago, IL, USA

Carmel Mallia, MD, FRCP (Lond., Edin.) Department of Medicine, Faculty of Medicine and Surgery, University of Malta, Msida, Malta

Marilyn Rogers, MD, MRCP (UK) Department of Medicine, Mater Dei Hospital, Msida, Malta

Chapter 1
Understanding Rheumatoid Arthritis

Carmel Mallia and Bernard Coleiro

1.1 Introduction

It is a misconception to think of or refer to rheumatoid arthritis simply as "arthritis". This is a mistake commonly made by laypersons who when asked if they suffer from any condition, they answer by saying "I suffer from arthritis" without specifying which type of arthritis. English literature also tends to reflect the same mistake, and we often come across narrative references to walking sticks implying the fictional character has "arthritis". English literature also tends to synonymously associate arthritis with old age. However, this is not always the case. The first thing to note about rheumatoid arthritis is that there are different types of arthritis and not all are strictly associated with old age. Certain types of arthritis can occur in younger patients, even in children.

The word "arthritis" is derived from Latin-Greek "arthron" meaning joint. Arthritis is a broad umbrella term used for conditions involving the joints and can be simplified into three distinct types of arthritis: namely, noninflammatory arthritis, inflammatory arthritis and metabolic arthritis. An example of noninflammatory arthritis would be osteoarthritis which is a degenerative old-age condition associated with wear and tear of the joints. Metabolic arthritis covers, on the other hand, conditions associated with deposition of crystals in joints, such as gout.

Rheumatoid arthritis, psoriatic arthritis, spondyloarthropathies and juvenile idiopathic arthritis are examples of inflammatory types of arthritis. Rheumatoid

---

C. Mallia, MD, FRCP (Lond., Edin.) (✉)
Department of Medicine, Faculty of Medicine and Surgery, University of Malta, Msida, Malta
e-mail: carmel.mallia@outlook.com

B. Coleiro, MD, FRCP, MPhil (Melit) (✉)
Faculty of Medicine and Surgery, University of Malta, Msida, Malta

Department of Medicine, Mater Dei Hospital, Msida, Malta
e-mail: bernardcoleiro454@gmail.com

© Springer Science+Business Media Singapore 2016
L. Grech, A. Lau (eds.), *Pharmaceutical Care Issues of Patients with Rheumatoid Arthritis*, DOI 10.1007/978-981-10-1421-5_1

arthritis, which is the commonest form of inflammatory arthritis, can be defined as a chronic, and therefore long-term, autoimmune systemic inflammatory disorder that involves several joints and that may effect any adult age group. Joint inflammation causes pain, and persistence of inflammation is followed by joint destruction which, apart from perpetuating pain, also leads to limitation of the effected joint mobility which, in turn, has a negative impact on the quality of life of patients. This chapter aims to explain the principles of rheumatoid arthritis and sets the foundation of the book starting out with a background historical overview of rheumatoid arthritis described in medical history.

1.2   Historical Overview of Rheumatoid Arthritis: From Skeleton to Art

The skeletal remains of Egyptian mummies, the skeletal remains of North American Indians found in Tennessee dating back to 4500 BC, and the ruins found in Pompeii indicate that rheumatoid arthritis is a condition which has long existed [1, 2]. Earliest descriptions of rheumatoid arthritis are documented in the famous Ebers Papyrus in an Indian text called the Charaka Samhita in AD 123 and various medical notes by the Greek Hippocrates, the physician of Caesar, Scribonius and the medical adviser of emperor Constantine IX, Michael Psellus. The texts describe a disease characterised by swollen and painful joints targeting initially the hands and feet but which progresses to other joints of the body [1–3]. It is interesting to note that in 1783, a report by a medical commission set up by the Grand Master of the Order of the Knights of St. John during their stay in Malta makes reference to a patient who suffered from rheumatism in both arms: "For four months, the articulations and the back of the left hand have been swollen. There is loss of movement in this hand and atrophy of the arm. The wrist is powerless, the movements of the fingers imperfect and the shape of the hand altered" [4]. This disease being described could easily have been rheumatoid arthritis. However, it is generally accepted that the first clear description of rheumatoid arthritis came about in 1800, when a young French doctor, Augustin Jacob Landre-Beauvais, put forward a clear description of rheumatoid arthritis in a lecture entitled Goute Asthenique Primitive (primary asthenic gout) before the Paris Academy of Medicine [5, 6]. In 1805, in his paper "Nodosity of joints", John Haygarth, while describing the disease, clinically noted the increased occurrence in the female sex compared to the male sex [7]. In 1859, Sir Alfred Garrod, a London physician, introduced the clinical term "rheumatoid arthritis" which included polyarticular osteoarthritis. In 1886, Bannantyre put forward the first radiological description of the term rheumatoid arthritis as we know it today. Subsequently, in 1907 it was Sir Alfred Garrod's son, Archibald Garrod, who distinguished the term osteoarthritis from rheumatoid arthritis [8–10].

Rheumatoid arthritis has been featured in art many years before its first clinical description: first in paintings during the seventeenth century when the artists started painting more precisely the human body. "The Painter's Family" painted between

1620 and 1622 by Jacob Jordaens housed in the Museo del Prado, Madrid, shows distinctly features of rheumatoid arthritis in the hand where the right hand of the housemaid who is carrying a basket of fruit shows clear signs of swelling of the meta-carpophalangeal (MCP) and proximal interphalangeal joints (PIP) [11]. Two other paintings, the "Adoration of the Magi" (1628) and "The Miracle of St. Ignatius of Loyola" (1618) both by Rubens also depict rheumatoid arthritis hand deformities [12]. Rubens himself suffered from a form of arthritis which, some suspect, may have been rheumatoid arthritis [12]. However, Pierre-August Renoir (1841–1919) is probably the most famous artist who suffered from rheumatoid arthritis, having suffered from the condition for the last 25 years of his life. Photos of the artist at 71 years of age show clear rheumatoid arthritis ulnar deviations in hand deformities [13, 14].

1.3 Prevalence

Literature indicates that the worldwide prevalence of rheumatoid arthritis remains at a constant of approximately 0.5–1 % of the world population [15–20]. However, factors, such as geographical distribution and industrialised status of countries, tend to effect the range of prevalence across the continents and sometimes across countries [21, 22]. In Europe, literature documents a higher incidence of rheumatoid arthritis in northern European countries compared to southern European countries [23–26]. Studies carried out amongst American Indians show a higher prevalence ranging between 5.3 % (Pima Indians) and 6.3 % (Chippewa Indians) [27, 28]. A higher incidence is again documented in industrialised countries compared to developing countries and in urban areas compared to rural areas [29].

As with most of the autoimmune diseases, rheumatoid arthritis is more likely to occur in females than in males with a ratio of 3:1. However, sex difference in prevalence is higher in the young generation since with advancing old age, the sex ratio approaches equality [30]. Finally contrary to misconceptions, though the peak onset of rheumatoid arthritis is between the fourth and fifth decades of life, it can occur at any age and is therefore not a disease of old age in contrast to osteoarthritis [31].

1.4 Pathophysiology

Articulating bones are covered with the articular cartilage which acts as a natural shock absorber by decreasing the friction between the bones as they move against each other. They are separated by the synovial cavity and are surrounded by an articular capsule. The articular capsule is composed of an outer layer called the fibrous capsule consisting of a dense irregular connective tissue and an inner layer called the synovial membrane. The synovial membrane consists of two layers: the subintima, consisting of connective tissue, elastic fibres and adipose tissue, and the intima, a thin sheet of cells that secretes synovial fluid made up of phagocytic cells and interstitial fluid formed from blood plasma into the synovial cavity. The synovial fluid reduces friction in the joint, supplies nutrients and removes debris resulting from wear and tear of the joint.

In rheumatoid arthritis the synovial membrane becomes persistently inflamed, leading to synovitis through angiogenesis and accumulation of synovial fluid in the synovial cavity. The inflammation clinically results in pain, swelling and warmth of the affected joint which, if sufficiently superficial, may also appear red. Inflammation in rheumatoid arthritis is triggered by an autoimmune reaction. Recent studies have shown that pro-inflammatory markers such as tumour necrosis factor (TNF) alpha, interleukin 6 (IL-6) and interleukin 1 (IL-1) are predominantly linked to the pathophysiology of rheumatoid arthritis [32–34]. At the cellular level, the synovial fluid becomes rich in inflammatory cells such as B cells, T cells, macrophages, plasma cells, polymorphonuclear leucocytes and pro-inflammatory cytokines [35, 36]. The role of the vascular endothelial growth factor (VEGF) in angiogenesis in rheumatoid arthritis is also implicated in association with the pathogenesis of rheumatoid arthritis, but further studies are required to better understand the role of VEGF in rheumatoid arthritis [37–39].

The persistent inflammation leads to a cascade of damage resulting in the formation of an abnormally thick synovial membrane (pannus), which extends beyond its normal boundaries and over the joint cartilage while stimulating the release of enzymes which destroy the articular cartilage. Once the articular cartilage (shock absorber) is eroded, the abnormal synovial membrane extends into the exposed bone ends, causing further bone destruction (manifested as joint erosion on X-ray). Secondary changes in the joint capsule and ligaments result in varying degrees of joint deformity.

1.5 Aetiology

The exact aetiology of rheumatoid arthritis remains unclear though various factors are implicated in the onset, severity and prognosis of the disease [40–45]. The genetic predisposition towards the gene HLA-DRB1 and the HLA-DR4 cluster alleles is associated with an increased risk of developing rheumatoid arthritis and extra-articular manifestations of the disease [46–52]. Over the years, various infective agents such as the Epstein-Barr virus and cytomegalovirus and bacterial organisms such as *Mycoplasma* and *Yersinia* have also been implicated as increasing the susceptibility towards the development of rheumatoid arthritis [53–55]. Some authors have indicated a possible association between periodontal disease and increased susceptibility to rheumatoid arthritis [56–59]. Smoking is the environmental factor closely associated with the onset and severity of rheumatoid arthritis. In addition, recent literature indicates that smoking decreases the effect of methotrexate and tumour necrosis factor inhibitor drugs on disease progression [60–63]. The hormonal association between rheumatoid arthritis and oestrogen is probably the least understood even though it is clear that a link does exist, considering the high female to male ratio at a young age when oestrogen levels are at their highest. The use of oral contraception tablets has been noted to offer some protection and postpone development of rheumatoid arthritis in postmenopausal women [64–66].

1.6 Clinical Manifestations

Patients with rheumatoid arthritis generally present with pain and stiffness which are worse in the morning. Joint stiffness after inactivity is typical of inflammatory joint disease; it is usually most marked after periods of inactivity – the longest of which is sleeping at night. This feature is referred to as early morning stiffness. This is quite characteristic of rheumatoid and other forms of inflammatory arthritis in contrast to the pain and mild stiffness of osteoarthritis which tend to occur after periods of activity and therefore at the end of the day. The duration of morning stiffness correlates with the degree of inflammation and therefore with the severity of the disease. The pain and early morning stiffness may be accompanied by other signs of inflammation, namely, increased warmth, swelling of the joint due to hypertrophy of the synovial membrane and joint effusion and erythema characterising the traditional Latin description of inflammation, namely, dolor (pain), rubor (redness, erythema), calor (heat), tumour (swelling) and functio laesa (impaired function).

The onset of rheumatoid arthritis is generally insidious, but sporadic cases of acute onset rarely occur. Rheumatoid arthritis can affect any joint sparing the vertebral joints and this is in contrast to spondyloarthropathies. Rheumatoid arthritis, which is symmetrical, commonly affects the hands and, if left untreated, results in the typical joint deformities that may include ulnar deviation of the fingers and Z deformity of the thumb. These deformities lead to diminished function of the hand leading to impairment of the quality of life of patients [67, 68].

Besides the clinical picture of the presenting complaint, rheumatoid arthritis is frequently associated with extra-articular manifestations and co-morbidities that result in death. Healthcare providers must be aware of these extra-articular manifestations and possibly aim at preventing their development. Extra-articular manifestations include anorexia, weight loss, malaise, lethargy, myalgia and low-grade fever [69]. These symptoms are very non-specific and can be easily missed. Besides, these are symptoms which are highly indicative of potential malignancies and must, therefore, be taken seriously. Rheumatoid arthritis can however cause more specific extra-articular manifestations in relation to organs [70–72].

1.6.1 Skin Manifestations, Oral and Ocular Involvement

Skin extra-articular manifestations associated with rheumatoid arthritis include rheumatoid nodules, which are mainly found on the extensor surface of the forearm. Rheumatoid arthritis may be accompanied by inflammation of blood vessels (vasculitis), and when this occurs, it tends to affect small blood vessels in the skin. Raynaud's phenomenon resulting due to spasm of the digital arteries is another unusual complication of rheumatoid arthritis, which can lead to ulceration and superinfection of the digits involved [73–77].

Sjogren's syndrome (also known as sicca – dry – syndrome), secondary to rheumatoid arthritis, can manifest itself via ocular and oral symptoms characterised by dry, gritty eyes with slight redness but normal vision and a dry mouth. Scleritis, which is another feature of rheumatoid arthritis, develops with severe pain with blurred vision and diffuse or nodular redness. A very rare complication of scleritis may lead to scleral thinning, secondary glaucoma and scleromalacia. Episcleritis, on the other hand, is a benign self-limiting condition where there is ocular irritation, redness and pain but without involvement of vision [78].

1.6.2 Pulmonary Manifestations

Pulmonary extra-articular manifestations associated with rheumatoid arthritis include pleuritis, pulmonary arteritis, pulmonary fibrosis and rarely Caplan's syndrome as well as obliterative bronchiolitis commonly known as bronchiolitis obliterans organising pneumonia (BOOP) [79–82].

1.6.3 Neurological Manifestations

Extra-articular features in relation to neurological involvement, which can occur secondary to rheumatoid arthritis, result mainly from the ongoing inflammatory process. These usually lead to central and peripheral compression syndromes such as carpal tunnel syndrome and nerve entrapment, as well as compression of the spinal cord resulting from subluxation of the articulation between the first two cervical vertebrae, the atlas and the axis (atlantoaxial subluxation) [83]. A mild form of peripheral neuropathy, predominantly sensory, may also occur in rheumatoid arthritis.

1.6.4 Renal Manifestations

Renal extra-articular manifestations are a cause of increased mortality and morbidity in rheumatoid arthritis patients. Glomerulonephritis, amyloidosis, acute or chronic interstitial nephritis and vasculitis have all been documented as renal involvement in rheumatoid arthritis patients [84–87]. Renal damage may also be caused by some of the medications that are used in the treatment of rheumatoid arthritis.

1.6.5   Felty's Syndrome

Felty's syndrome is a condition where rheumatoid arthritis is associated with splenomegaly and neutropenia in addition to hepatomegaly and lymphadenopathy. It may be associated with serious infections, vasculitis of skin blood vessels leading to leg ulcers and vasculitis of the small blood vessels supplying nerves (vasa nervorum) leading to mononeuritis multiplex. Anaemia and thrombocytopenia may also occur and increase the risk of mortality and morbidity. Felty's syndrome is strongly associated with the presence of a strongly positive rheumatoid factor, a positive anti-nuclear antibody (ANA) and a positive HLA-DR4*0401 antigen [88].

1.6.6   Cardiovascular Co-morbidities and Rheumatoid Arthritis

There is a fine line between extra-articular features and co-morbidities when it comes to discussing cardiovascular disease. Indeed, cardiovascular disease is a common co-morbidity in rheumatoid arthritis, and studies indicate that it is most likely responsible for increased mortality and morbidity when compared to the general population [89–92]. Evidence suggests that an increased accumulation of oxidised low-density lipoprotein is seen in rheumatoid arthritis patients [93–95]. This is a risk factor for coronary heart disease. Due to increasing evidence of the link between cardiovascular disease and rheumatoid arthritis, in 2010 the European League Against Rheumatism (EULAR) felt that it was opportune to publish evidence-based recommendations for cardiovascular risk management in patients with rheumatoid arthritis [96].

1.6.7   Malignancy

The persistent ongoing inflammatory process to which rheumatoid arthritis patients are subjected may result in an increased risk of developing solid tumour, skin and haematological malignancies [97, 98].

1.6.8   Osteoporosis

The relationship between osteoporosis and rheumatoid arthritis is the result of a number of factors including disease-related immobility, the increased occurrence of rheumatoid arthritis in female population compared to the male population, the intermittent steroid therapy and the production of pro-inflammatory cytokines such as interleukins and tumour necrosis factors which are implicated in bone resorption [99, 100].

1.7 Relevant Investigations

There is no laboratory investigation which is specific to rheumatoid arthritis and which can therefore be said to be diagnostic of rheumatoid arthritis. All relevant laboratory investigations need to be taken in consideration together with the clinical picture with which the patient presents.

Relevant investigations within rheumatoid arthritis can be classified as laboratory investigations and radiological imaging. Both investigations serve two main aims: first to aid clinicians confirm the diagnosis and second to assess disease activity and response to pharmacotherapy prescribed. Table 1.1 summarises suggested relevant laboratory investigations.

Radiological images such as X-ray images, ultrasound images and magnetic resonance images (MRI) of the effected joint/s can help confirm diagnosis of rheumatoid arthritis [101]. During the course of rheumatoid arthritis, such images can detect progression of the disease and also aid in delivering direct infiltrations of anti-inflammatory medication such as steroids as close and as precise as possible to the effected joint. However, it is important to note that X-ray changes in rheumatoid arthritis, the typical of which being joint erosions, are late to appear. In fact, these take approximately 2 years after onset of the disease before becoming apparent. On the other hand, the more modern methods of imaging joints, such as ultrasound and MRI scans, are much more sensitive and show damage at a much earlier stage of the disease, hence their usefulness in diagnosing the disease in its early stages.

1.8 Diagnosis of Rheumatoid Arthritis

The diagnosis of rheumatoid arthritis is mostly based on the clinical features manifested by the patient. In the absence of specific markers to pin down the diagnosis of rheumatoid arthritis, the clinicians very often rely on the classification criteria for rheumatoid arthritis. The 2010 ACR/EULAR classification criteria for rheumatoid arthritis which was jointly put forward by the American College of Rheumatology (ACR) and the European League Against Rheumatism (EULAR) are currently in use [102]. The new criteria incorporate joint assessment, two serology assessments and duration of symptoms. It has been validated to capture early rheumatoid arthritis [103]. Table 1.2 represents the 2010 ACR/EULAR classification criteria for rheumatoid arthritis. In addition to the tests put forward in the 2010 ACR/EULAR classification criteria for rheumatoid arthritis, clinicians can easily perform the squeeze test also known as Gaenslen's test. This consists of compression of the metacarpophalangeal (MCP) or metatarsophalangeal (MTP) joints to elicit pain in response to inflammation secondary to rheumatoid arthritis. It is a cheap, easy and non-invasive method which can help clinicians detect synovitis linked to inflammation in early rheumatoid arthritis [104–106].

Table 1.1 Suggested laboratory investigations

Test	Clinical relevance	Interpretation in rheumatoid arthritis
C-reactive protein (CRP)	Tests the level of CRP, an acute phase reactant protein produced by the liver following inflammation Venous sample is taken	High It rises soon after the inflammatory cascade is triggered and subsequently decreases fast once the inflammation settles
Erythrocyte sedimentation rate (ESR)	Tests the rate at which the erythrocytes sediment from a sample of blood over 1 h. In the presence of acute phase reactant proteins, the erythrocytes sediment more rapidly Venous sample in a specific standard bottle	High
Complete blood count (CBC)	Evaluates: i. The white blood cells giving the number of neutrophils, lymphocytes, basophils, eosinophils and monocytes ii. The red blood cells giving the number of erythrocytes, the haemoglobin level, haematocrit, mean corpuscular volume (MCV), mean corpuscular haemoglobin (MCH), the mean corpuscular haemoglobin concentration (MCHC) and the red cell width distribution iii. The platelets giving the platelet count Venous sample is taken	Anaemia and thrombocytosis are common in active rheumatoid arthritis Drug profile can interfere with CBC
Rheumatoid factor (RF)	Tests the serum level of the antibody for immunoglobulin M (IgM) in the blood Venous sample taken but serum worked out	May be positive or negative A positive result against clinical rheumatoid arthritis features indicates poorer prognosis
Anti-cyclic citrullinated peptide (anti-CCP)	Tests the serum level of the antibodies against cyclic citrillunated peptide. Cyclic citrullinated peptide is present at a higher rate in inflammation of the joints. Can be detected in early RA disease Venous sample is taken	A positive result in the absence of clinical features of rheumatoid arthritis indicates a high risk for developing rheumatoid arthritis High levels at diagnosis indicate aggressive disease and poorer prognosis
Anti-nuclear antibody (ANA)	Tests the serum level of anti-nuclear antibodies which are autoantibodies produced by the immune system Venous sample is taken	Can be positive or negative It is more highly indicative of systemic lupus erythematosus

Table 1.2 2010 ACR/EULAR classification criteria for rheumatoid arthritis

Domain	Definition	Score
A. Joint involvement		
1 large joint	Shoulder, elbows, hips, knees, ankles	0
2–10 large joints		1
1–3 small joints ± involvement of large joints	Small joints: metacarpophalangeal joints, proximal interphalangeal joints, second to fifth metatarsophalangeal joints, thumb, interphalangeal joints, wrists	2
4–10 small joints ± involvement of large joints		3
>10 joints with at least one small joint	One small joint involvement and any other joints	5
B. Serology		
Negative RF and negative anti-CCP	Negative levels are equal to or less than the normal value. Low positive levels are defined as levels higher than normal level but which are three times less than the normal upper limit. High positive values are defined as levels which are three times more than the normal upper limit	0
Low positive RF or low positive anti-CCP		2
High positive RF or high positive anti-CCP		3
C. Acute phase reactants		
Normal CRP + normal ESR		0
Abnormal CRP or normal ESR		1
D. Duration of symptoms		
<6 weeks		0
>6 weeks		1

A total score equal to or more than six indicates definite rheumatoid arthritis. A score less than six does not indicate current rheumatoid arthritis, but it does not exclude that the patient might later on develop rheumatoid arthritis

1.9 Pregnancy and Breastfeeding

In general, unlike systemic lupus erythematosus, rheumatoid arthritis tends to be quiescent during pregnancy, and most of the flare-ups tend to occur post-partum [107]. Clinically, this is a good aspect since pregnancy limits the use of potentially effective drugs such as methotrexate, leflunomide and biological drugs.

On the other hand, the post-partum period is also associated with a higher incidence of onset of rheumatoid arthritis [108]. Breastfeeding in rheumatoid arthritis mothers has been associated with increased flare-ups possibly due to increased secretion of the hormone prolactin during breastfeeding [109–111].

1.10   Early Diagnosis: A Must to Ensure Better Prognosis and Improved Quality of Life

Rheumatoid arthritis is a chronic, progressive autoimmune disease leading to joint destruction which, if untreated, results in deformities, extra-articular manifestations leading to impaired quality of life and impacting on patients' activities of daily living [112]. The crucial point is therefore early detection of symptoms indicative of the condition, early confirmation of the diagnosis of rheumatoid arthritis and early initiation of treatment to slow down disease progression as much as possible, limiting joint destruction and affording a better prognosis [113–117]. Nowadays, the diagnosis of early rheumatoid arthritis is possible through the combination of clinical features and appropriate and timely investigations, including the use of ultrasonography and magnetic resonance imaging which, as already stated, are very sensitive to detect joint damage at an early stage of the disease [118–121]. Clinically the earlier the diagnosis is made and the earlier the treatment is started, the better the prognosis and the better the eventual quality of life of the rheumatoid arthritis patient. In a real case scenario, treatment should be started within 12 weeks since presentation of the patient in order to expect the best possible outcome [101, 122].

Take-Home Messages
- Rheumatoid arthritis is a chronic (long-term) autoimmune systemic inflammatory condition of the joints, affecting any age group and which if left untreated will result in pain, joint deformities and co-morbidities severely impacting the patients' quality of life leading to overall added socio-economic constraints.
- It is strongly associated with extra-articular manifestations and co-morbidities of which cardiovascular disease is the most common.
- Female to male ratio is 3:1 but it approaches equality with advancing age.
- Diagnosis is heavily based on the clinical picture with the aid of serological markers.
- The anti-cyclic citrullinated peptide (anti-CCP) antibody is a good marker for detection of early rheumatoid arthritis.
- Rheumatoid arthritis tends to calm down during pregnancy.
- Early diagnosis of rheumatoid arthritis leads to early treatment resulting in better prognosis and improved quality of life of patients.

Famous People Who Suffered from Rheumatoid Arthritis

British scientist *Dorothy Hodgkin* (1910–1994) developed X-ray crystallography for the identification of 3D structures of biological molecules such as penicillin, insulin and vitamin B12. Hodgkin went on to win the 1964 Nobel Prize for Chemistry. She died at the age of 84 having suffered from rheumatoid arthritis since approximately the age of 24.

Edith Piaf (1915–1963) was a French singer who rose to fame during World War II. She developed rheumatoid arthritis at 34 years and died aged 47 due to liver cancer. Two of her famous songs include *"La Vie en Rose"* (1946) and *"Non, Je ne Regrette Rien"* (1960). Later on, a biographic movie entitled *"La Vie en Rose"* (2007) was produced and depicts amongst others Piaf's struggle with rheumatoid arthritis.

Dr. Christiaan Barnard (1922–2001) a South African cardiac surgeon who in 1967 performed the first human-to-human heart transplant procedure. Though the patient died 18 days after surgery, this was the first such operation. Dr. Barnard developed rheumatoid arthritis at the age of 34. Subsequently in 1983 he developed hand deformities which led him to retire from his career. Eventually, he wrote a book on coping with arthritis.

Hollywood actor *James Coburn* (1928–2002) featured in over 70 movies amongst which "The Magnificent Seven" and "The Great Escape". In 1979 aged 51 years, he was diagnosed with rheumatoid arthritis which saw him cut out on his career as an actor but reappeared in the 1990s in supporting acts in various movies such as *Sister Act 2* and *The Nutty Professor*. In 1998, Coburn won the Academy Award for Best Supporting Actor for his role in the movie "Affliction".

References

1. Entezami P, Fox DA, Clapham PJ, Chung KC (2011) Historical perspective on the aetiology of rheumatoid arthritis. Hand Clin 27(1):1–10
2. Joshi VR (2012) Rheumatology, past, present and future. JAPI 60:21–24
3. Deshpande S (2014) History of rheumatology. Med J Dr DY Patil Univ 7(2):119–123
4. Cassar P (1964) Medical History of Malta. Publications of the Wellcome Historical Medical Library. New Series Vol. VI. General Editor FNL Poynyter
5. Landre-Beauvais AJ (2001) The first correct description of rheumatoid arthritis. Unabridged text of the doctoral dissertation presented in 1800. Joint Bone Spine 68(2):130–143
6. Parish LC (1963) An historical approach to the nomenclature of rheumatoid arthritis. Arthritis Rheum 6(2):138–158
7. Booth C (2015) John Haygarth: a physician of the enlightenment. American Philosophical Society, Philadelphia
8. Short CL (1974) The antiquity of rheumatoid arthritis. Arthritis Rheum 17(3):193–205
9. Mallia C (2004) Treating rheumatoid arthritis, yesterday and today. MMJ 16(2):18–21
10. Bannatyne G, Wohlmann A (1896) Rheumatoid arthritis: its clinical history, etiology, pathology. Lancet 147(3791):1120–1125
11. Dequeker J (1977) Arthritis in Flemish paintings. Br Med J 1(6070):1203–1205

12. Appelboom T (2005) Hypothesis: Rubens – one of the first victims of an epidemic of rheumatoid arthritis that started in the 16th-17th century? Rheumatology 44:681–683
13. Boonen A, van de Rest J, Dequeker J, van der Linden S (1997) How Renoir coped with rheumatoid arthritis. BMJ 315:1705
14. Kowalski E, Chung KC (2012) Impairment and disability: Renoir's adaptive coping strategies with rheumatoid arthritis. Hand 7:357–363
15. Hochberg MC (1981) Adult and juvenile rheumatoid arthritis: current epidemiologic concepts. Epidemiol Rev 3:27
16. Silman AJ (1998) Epidemiology and the rheumatic diseases. In: Maddison PJ, Isenberg DA, Woo P, Glass DN (eds) Oxford textbook of rheumatology. Oxford University Press, Oxford, p 506
17. Gabriel SE (2001) The epidemiology of rheumatoid arthritis. Rheum Dis Clin North Am 27(2):269–281
18. Silman AJ, Hochberg MC (2001) Rheumatoid arthritis. In: Silman AJ, Hochberg MC (eds) Epidemiology of the rheumatic diseases. Oxford University Press, Oxford, pp 31–71
19. Alamanos Y, Drosos AA (2005) Epidemiology of adult rheumatoid arthritis. Autoimmun Rev 4(3):130–136
20. Gibofsky A (2014) Epidemiology, pathophysiology and diagnosis of rheumatoid arthritis: a synopsis. Am J Manag Care 20(Suppl 7):S128–S135
21. Silman AJ, Pearson JE (2002) Epidemiology and genetics of rheumatoid arthritis. Arthritis Res 4(Suppl 3):S265–S272
22. Woolf AD, Pfleger B (2003) Burden of major musculoskeletal conditions. Bull World Health Organ 81(9):646–656
23. Guillemin F, Saraux A, Guggenbuhl P, Roux CH, Fardellone P, Le Bihan E, Cantagrel A et al (2005) Prevalence of rheumatoid arthritis in France: 2001. Ann Rheum Dis 64:1427–1430
24. Alamanos Y, Voulgari PV, Drosos AA (2006) Incidence and prevalence of rheumatoid arthritis, based on the 1987 American College of Rheumatology criteria: a systematic review. Semin Arthritis Rheum 36(3):182–188
25. Carbonell J, Cobo T, Balsa A, Descalzo MA, Carmona L (2008) The incidence of rheumatoid arthritis in Spain: results from a nationwide primary care registry. Rheumatology 47(7):1088–1092
26. Pedersen JK, Kjaer NK, Svendsen AJ, Horslev-Petersen K (2009) Incidence of rheumatoid arthritis from 1995 to 2001: impact of ascertainment from multiple sources. Rheumatol Int 29(4):411–415
27. Harvey J, Lotze M, Stevens MB, Lambert G, Jacobson D (1981) Rheumatoid arthritis in a Chippewa band. I Pilot screening study of disease prevalence. Arthritis Rheum 24:717–721
28. Del Puente A, Knowler WC, Pettit DJ, Bennett PH (1989) High incidence and prevalence of rheumatoid arthritis in Pima Indians. Am J Epidemiol 129:1170–1178
29. Tobon GJ, Youinou P, Saraux A (2010) The environment, geo-epidemiology and autoimmune disease: rheumatoid arthritis. Autoimmun Rev 9(5):A288–A292
30. Akil M, Veerapen K (2004) Rheumatoid arthritis: clinical features and diagnosis. In: Snaith ML (ed) ABC of rheumatology. BMJ, London, pp 50–55
31. Markenson JA (1991) Worldwide trends in the socioeconomic impact and long term prognosis of rheumatoid arthritis. Semin Arthritis Rheum 21(Suppl 1):4–12
32. Smolen JS, Steiner G (2003) Therapeutic strategies for rheumatoid arthritis. Nat Rev Drug Discov 2:473–488
33. McInness IB, Schett G (2007) Cytokines in the pathogenesis of rheumatoid arthritis. Nat Rev Immunol 7:429–442
34. Smolen JS, Aletaha D, Koeller M, Weisman MH, Emery P (2007) New therapies for treatment of rheumatoid arthritis. Lancet 370:1861–1874
35. Choy E (2012) Understanding the dynamics: pathways involved in the pathogenesis of rheumatoid arthritis. Rheumatology 51(S5):v3–v11

36. Cooles FAH, Isaacs JD (2011) Pathophysiology of rheumatoid arthritis. Curr Opin Rheumatol 2393:233–240
37. Koch AE (2000) The role of angiogenesis in rheumatoid arthritis:recent developments. Ann Rheum Dis 59(Suppl I):65–71
38. Taylor P (2002) VEGF and imaging of vessels in rheumatoid arthritis. Arthritis Res 4(Suppl 3):S99–S107
39. de Bandt M, Ben Mahdi MH, Ollivier V, Grossin M, Dupuis M, Gaudry M et al (2003) Blockade of vascular endothelial growth factor receptor-1 (VEGF-RI) but not VEGF-RII, suppresses joint destruction in the K/BxN model of rheumatoid arthritis. J Immunol 171:4853–4859
40. Carlens C, Jacobsson L, Brandt L, Cranttingius O, Stephansson O, Askling J (2009) Perinatal characteristics, early life infections and later risk of rheumatoid arthritis and juvenile idiopathic arthritis. Ann Rheum Dis 68:1159–1164
41. van der Helm-van Mil AHM, Toes REM, Huizinga TWJ (2010) Genetic variants in the prediction of rheumatoid arthritis. Ann Rheum Dis 69:1694–1696
42. van de Sande MGH, de Hair MJH, van der Leij C, Klarenbeek PL, Bos WH, Smith MD et al (2011) Different stages of rheumatoid arthritis: features of the synovium in the preclinical phase. Ann Rheum Dis 70:772–777
43. Scott IC, Steer S, Lewis CM, Cope AP (2011) Precipitating and perpetuating factors of rheumatoid arthritis immunopathology: linking the triad of genetic predisposition, environmental risk factors and autoimmunity to disease pathogenesis. Best Pract Res Clin Rheumatol 25:447–468
44. de Hair MJH, Landewe RBM, van de Sande MGH, van Schaardenburg D, van Baarsen LGM, Gerlag DM et al (2012) Smoking and overweight determine the likelihood of developing rheumatoid arthritis. Ann Rheum Dis 72:1654–1658
45. Lundberg K, Bengtsson C, Kharlamova N, Reed R, Jiang X, Kallberg H et al (2013) Genetic and environmental determinants for disease risk in subsets of rheumatoid arthritis defined by the anticitrullinated protein/peptide antibody fine specificity profile. Ann Rheum Dis 72:652–658
46. Ruiz-Morales JA, Vargas-Alarcon G, Flores-Villanueva PO, Villarreal-Garza C, Hernandez-Pacheco G, Yamamoto-Furusho JK et al (2004) HLA-DRB1 alleles encoding the "shared epitope" are associated with susceptibility to developing rheumatoid arthritis whereas HLA-DRB1 alleles encoding an aspartic acid at position 70 of the beta-chain are protective in Mexican Mestizos. Human Immunol 65(3):262–269
47. Barnetche T, Constantin A, Cantagrel A, Cambon-Thomsen A, Gourraud PA (2008) New classification of HLA-DRB1 alleles in rheumatoid arthritis susceptibility: a combined analysis of worldwide samples. Arthritis Res Ther 10(1):R26
48. Morgan AW, Haroon-Rashid L, Martin SG, Gooi HC, Worthington J, Thomson W et al (2008) The shared epitope hypothesis in rheumatoid arthritis: evaluation of alternative classification criteria in a large UK Caucasian cohort. Arthritis Rheum 58(5):1275–1283
49. Barton A, Worthington J (2009) Genetic susceptibility to rheumatoid arthritis: an emerging picture. Arthritis Rheum 61(10):1441–1446
50. Holoshitz J (2010) The rheumatoid arthritis HLA-DRB1 shared epitope. Curr Opin Rheumatol 22(3):293–298
51. Reynolds RJ, Ahmed AF, Danila MI, Hughes LB, Consortium for the Longitudinal Evaluation of African Americans with Early Rheumatoid Arthritis et al (2014) HLA-DRB1-associated rheumatoid arthritis risk at multiple levels in African Americans: hierarchical classification systems, amino acid positions and residues. Arthritis Rheumatol 66(12):3271–3282
52. Louthrenoo W, Kasitanon N, Wangkaew S, Kuwata S, Takeuchi F (2015) Distribution of HLA-DR alleles among Thai patients with rheumatoid arthritis. Human Immunol 76(2–3):113–117
53. Alspaugh MA, Henle G, Lennette ET, Henle W (1981) Elevated levels of antibodies to Epstein Barr virus antigens in sera and synovial fluids of patients with rheumatoid arthritis. J Clin Invest 67:1134–1140

54. Cohen BJ, Buckley MM, Clewley JP, Jones VE, Puttick AH, Jacoby RK (1986) Human parvovirus infection in early rheumatoid and inflammatory arthritis. Ann Rheum Dis 45:832–838
55. Buch M, Emery P (2002) The aetiology and pathogenesis of rheumatoid arthritis. Hosp Pharm 9:5–10
56. Greenwald RA, Kirkwood K (1999) Adult periodontitis as model for rheumatoid arthritis (with emphasis on treatment strategies). J Rheumatol 26:1650–1653
57. Rosentein ED, Greenwald RA, Kushner LJ, Weissmann G (2004) Hypothesis: the humoral immune response to oral bacteria provides a stimulus for the development of rheumatoid arthritis. Inflammation 28:311–318
58. Hitchon CA, Chandad F, Ferucci ED et al (2010) Antibodies to porphyromonas gingivalis are associated with anticitrullinated protein antibodies in patients with rheumatoid arthritis and their relatives. J Rheumatol 37(6):1105–1112
59. Routsias JG, Goules JD, Goules A, Charalampakis G, Pikazis D (2011) Autopathogenic correlation of periodontitis and rheumatoid arthritis. Rheumatology 50(7):1189–1193
60. Sugiyama D, Nishimura K, Tamaki K, Tsuji G, Nakazawa T, Morinobu A et al (2010) Impact of smoking as a risk factor for developing rheumatoid arthritis: a meta-analysis of observational studies. Ann Rheum Dis 69:70–81
61. Saevarsdottir S, Wedren S, Seddighzadeh M, Bengtsson C, Wesley A, Lindblad S et al (2011) Patients with early rheumatoid arthritis who smoke are less likely to respond to treatment with methotrexate and tumour necrosis factor inhibitors: observations from the Epidemiological Investigation of Rheumatoid Arthritis and the Swedish Rheumatology Register cohorts. Arthritis Rheum 63(1):26–36
62. Soderlin MK, Petersson IF, Geborek P (2012) The effect of smoking on response and drug survival in rheumatoid arthritis patients treated with their first anti-TNF drug. Scand J Rheumatol 41(1):1–9
63. Chang K, Yang SM, Kim SH, Han KH, Park SJ, Shin JI (2014) Smoking and rheumatoid arthritis. Int J Mol Sci 15(12):22279–22295
64. Brennan P, Bankhead C, Silman A, Symmons D (1997) Oral contraceptives and rheumatoid arthritis: results from primary care-based incident case control study. Semin Arthritis Rheum 26:817–823
65. Hannaford PC, Kay CR, Hirsch S (1990) Oral contraceptives and rheumatoid arthritis: new data from the Royal College of General Practitioners' oral contraception study. Ann Rheum Dis 49:744–746
66. Cutolo M, Capellino S, Straub RH (2008) Oestrogens in rheumatic diseases: friend or foe? Rheumatology 47(S3):2–5
67. Chung KC, Pushman AG (2011) Current concepts in the management of the rheumatoid hand. J Hand Surg Am 36(4):736–747
68. Malahias M, Gardner H, Hindocha S, Juma A, Khan W (2012) The future of rheumatoid arthritis and hand surgery – combining evolutionary pharmacology and surgical technique. Open Orthop J 6:88–94
69. Young A, Koduri G (2007) Extra-articular manifestations and complications of rheumatoid arthritis. Best Pract Res Clin Rheumatol 21(5):907–927
70. Turesson C, O'Fallon WM, Crowson CS, Gabriel SE, Matteson EL (2003) Extra-articular disease manifestations in rheumatoid arthritis: incidence trends and risk factors over 46 years. Ann Rheum Dis 62:722–727
71. Mjelants H, van den Bosch F (2009) Extra-articular manifestations. Clin Exp Rheumatol 27:S56–S61
72. Cojocaru M, Cojocaru IM, Silosi I, Vrabie CD, Tanasescu R (2010) Extra-articular manifestations in rheumatoid arthritis. Maedica (Buchar) 54(4):286–291
73. Sayah A, English JC (2005) Rheumatoid arthritis: a review of the cutaneous manifestations. J Am Acad Dermatol 53(2):191–209
74. Genta MS, Genta RM, Gabay C (2006) Systemic rheumatoid vasculitis: a review. Semin Arthritis Rheum 36(2):88–98

75. Marzano AV (2013) Cutaneous manifestations in rheumatoid arthritis. Clin Dermatol 1(2):53–59
76. Bartels CM, Bridges AJ (2010) Rheumatoid vasculitis: vanishing menace or target for new treatments? Curr Rheumatol Rep 12(6):414–419
77. Makol A, Matteson E, Warrington KJ (2015) Rheumatoid vasculitis: an update. Curr Opin Rheumatol 27(1):63–70
78. Artifoni M, Rothschild PR, Brezin A, Guillevin L, Peuchal X (2014) Ocular inflammatory diseases associated with rheumatoid arthritis. Nat Rev Rheumatol 10(2):108–116
79. Ippolito JA, Palmer L, Spector S, Kane PB, Gorevic PD (1993) Bronchiolitis obliterans organizing pneumonia and rheumatoid arthritis. Semin Arthritis Rheum 23(1):70–78
80. Schreiber J, Koschel D, Kekow J, Waldburg N, Goette A, Merget R (2010) Rheumatoid pneumoconiosis (Caplan's syndrome). Eur J Intern Med 21(3):168–172
81. O'Dwyer DN, Armstrong ME, Cooke G, Dood JD, Veale DJ, Donnelly SC (2013) Rheumatoid arthritis associated interstitial lung disease. Eur J Intern Med 24(7):597–603
82. Kelly CA, Saravanan V, Nisar M, Arthanari S, Woodhead FA, Price-Forbes AN et al (2014) Rheumatoid arthritis-related interstitial lung disease: associations, prognostic factors and physiological and radiological characteristics – a large multicenter UK study. Rheumatology 53(9):1676–1682
83. Ramos-Remus C, Duran-Barragan S, Castillo-Ortiz JD (2012) Beyond the joints: neurological involvement in rheumatoid arthritis. Clin Rheumatol 3(11):1–12
84. Icardi A, Araghi P, Ciabattoni M, Romano U, Lazzarini P, Bianchi G (2003) Kidney involvement in rheumatoid arthritis. Reumatismo 55(2):76–85
85. Karie S, Gandjbakhch F, Janus N, Launay-Vacher V, Rozenberg S, Mai Ba CU et al (2008) Kidney disease in rheumatoid arthritis patients: prevalence and implications of RA-related drugs management: the MATRIX study. Rheumatology 47(3):350–354
86. Anders HJ, Vielhauer V (2011) Renal co-morbidity in patients with rheumatic disease. Arthritis Res Ther 13:222
87. Kranbichler A, Mayer G (2013) Renal involvement in autoimmune connective tissue disease. BMC Med 11:95
88. Balint GP, Balint PV (2004) Felty's syndrome. Best Pract Res Clin Rheumatol 18(5):631–645
89. Wolfe F, Freundich B, Straus WL (2003) Increase in cardiovascular and cerebrovascular disease prevalence in rheumatoid arthritis. J Rheumatol 30:36–40
90. Kitas GD, Gabriel SE (2011) Cardiovascular disease in rheumatoid arthritis: state of the art and future perspectives. Ann Rheum Dis 70:8–14
91. Choy E, Ganeshalingam K, Semb AG, Szekanecz Z, Nurmohamed M (2014) Cardiovascular risk in rheumatoid arthritis: recent advances in the understanding of the pivotal role of inflammation, risk predictors and the impact of treatment. Rheumatology 53(12):2143–2154
92. Dougados M, Soubrier M, Antunez A, Balint P, Balsa A, Buch M et al (2014) Prevalence of comorbidities of rheumatoid arthritis and evaluation of their monitoring. Results from an international cross-sectional study, COMORA. Ann Rheum Dis 73(1):62–68
93. Myasoedova E, Crownson CS, Kremers HM, Roger VL, Fitz-Gibbon PD, Therneau TM et al (2011) Lipid paradox in rheumatoid arthritis: the impact of serum lipid measures and systemic inflammation on the risk of cardiovascular disease. Ann Rheum Dis 70(3):482–487
94. Robertston J, Peters MJ, McInnes IB, Sattar N (2013) Changes in lipid levels with inflammation and therapy in RA: a maturing paradigm. Nat Rev Rheumatol 9(9):513–523
95. Zhang J, Chen L, Delzell E, Muntner P, Hillegass WB, Safford MM et al (2014) The association between inflammatory markers, serum lipids and the risk of cardiovascular events in patients with rheumatoid arthritis. Ann Rheum Dis 73(7):1301–1308
96. Peters MJL, Symmons DPM, McCarey D, Dijkmans DAC, Nikola P, Kvien TK et al (2010) Eular evidence based recommendations for cardiovascular risk management in patients with rheumatoid arthritis and other forms of inflammatory arthritis. Ann Rheum Dis 69:325–331

97. Askling J (2007) Malignancy and rheumatoid arthritis. Curr Rheumatol Rep 9(5):421–426
98. Smitten A, Simon TA, Hochberg MC, Suissa S (2008) A meta-analysis of the incidence of malignancy in adult patients with rheumatoid arthritis. Arthritis Res Ther 10(2):R45
99. Sinigaglia L, Nervetti A, Mela Q, Bianchi G, del Puente A, Di Munno O et al (2000) A multicenter cross sectional study on bone mineral density in rheumatoid arthritis. Italian Study Group on Bone Mass in Rheumatoid Arthritis. J Rheumatol 27:2582–2589
100. McLean R (2009) Proinflammatory cytokines and osteoporosis. Curr Osteoporos Res 7:134–139
101. Smolen JS, Breedveld FC, Burmester G, Bykerk V, Dougados M, Emery P et al (2015) Treating rheumatoid arthritis to target: 2014 update of the recommendations of an international task force. Ann Rheum Dis 75:3–15. doi:10.1136/annrheumdis-2015.207524
102. Aletaha D, Neogi T, Silman AJ, Funovits J, Felson DT, Bingham CO (2010) Rheumatoid arthritis classification criteria: an American College of Rheumatology/European League against Rheumatism collaborative initiative. Ann Rheum Dis 2010(69):1580–1588
103. Humphreys JH, Verstappen SMM, Hyrich KL, Chipping JR, Marshall T, Symmons DPM (2012) The incidence of rheumatoid arthritis in the United Kingdom: comparisons using the 2010 ACR/EULAR classification criteria and the 1987 ACR classification criteria. Results from the Norfolk Arthritis Register. Ann Rheum Dis 00:1–6
104. Wiesinger T, Smolen JS, Aletaha D, Stamm T (2013) Compression test (Gaenslen's squeeze test) positivity, joint tenderness and disease activity in patients with rheumatoid arthritis. Arthritis Care Res 65(4):653–657
105. van den Bosch WB, Mangnus L, Reijnierse M, Huizinga TW, van der Helm-van Mil AH (2015) The diagnostic accuracy of the squeeze test to identify arthritis: a cross sectional cohort study. Ann Rheum Dis 74(10):1886–1889
106. Vega-Morales D, Esquivel-Valerio JA, Garza-Elizondo MA (2015) Do rheumatologists know how to squeeze? Evaluation of Gaenslen's maneuver. Rheumatol Int 35(12):2037–2040
107. Kanik KS, Wilder RL (2000) Hormonal alterations in rheumatoid arthritis, including the effects of pregnancy. Rheum Dis Clin North Am 26(4):805–823
108. Silman AJ, Kay A, Brennan P (1992) Timing of pregnancy in relation to the onset of rheumatoid arthritis. Arthritis Rheum 35:152–155
109. Brennan P, Hajeer A, Ong KR, Worthington J, John S, Thomson W, Silman A, Ollier B (1997) Allelic markers close to prolactin are associated with HLA-DRB1 susceptibility alleles among women with rheumatoid arthritis and systemic lupus erythematosus. Arthritis Rheum 40:1383–1386
110. Brennan P, Silman A (1994) Breastfeeding and the onset of rheumatoid arthritis. Arthritis Rheum 37:808–813
111. Olsen NJ, Kovacs WJ (2002) Hormones, pregnancy and rheumatoid arthritis. J Gend Specif Med 5(4):28–37
112. Cush JJ (2007) Early rheumatoid arthritis – is there a window of opportunity? Rheumatol Supp 80:1–7
113. Emery P, Breedveld FC, Dougados M, Kalden JR, Schiff MH, Smolen JS (2002) Early referral recommendation for newly diagnosed rheumatoid arthritis: evidence based development of a clinical guide. Ann Rheum Dis 61(4):290–297
114. Bosello S, Fedele AL, Peluso G, Gremese E, Tolusso B, Ferraccioli G (2011) Very early rheumatoid arthritis is the major predictor of major outcomes: clinical ACR remission and radiographic non-progression. Ann Rheum Dis 70(7):1292–1295
115. Feldman DE, Bernatsky S, Houde M, Beauchamp ME, Abrahamowicz M (2013) Early consultation with a rheumatologist for RA: does it reduce subsequent use of orthopaedic surgery? Rheumatology 52(3):452–459
116. Kyburz D, Finckh A (2013) The importance of early treatment for the prognosis of rheumatoid arthritis. Swiss Med Wkly 143:w13865
117. Raza K, Mallen CD (2013) Rheumatoid arthritis: what do we mean by early? Rheumatology 52(3):411–412

118. da Mota LM, Laurindo IMM, dos Santos Neto LL, Lima FA, Viana SL, Mendlovitz PS et al (2012) Imaging diagnosis of early rheumatoid arthritis. Rev Bras Rheumatol 52(5):757–766

119. Thiele RG (2012) Ultrasonography applications in diagnosis and management of early rheumatoid arthritis. Rheum Dis Clin North Am 38(2):259–275

120. Colebatch AN, Edwards CJ, Ostergaard M, van der Heijde D, Balint PV, D'Agostino MA et al (2013) EULAR recommendations for the use of imaging of the joints in the clinical management of rheumatoid arthritis. Ann Rheum Dis 72(6):804–814

121. Ten Cate DF, Luime JJ, Swen N, Gerards AH, De Jager MH, Basoski NM et al (2013) Role of ultrasonography in diagnosing early rheumatoid arthritis and remission of rheumatoid arthritis – a systematic review of the literature. Arthritis Res Ther 15(1):R4

122. Gremese E, Salaffi F, Bosello SL, Ciapetti A, Bobbio-Pallavicini F, Caporali R et al (2013) Very early rheumatoid arthritis as a predictor of remission: a multicentre real life prospective study. Ann Rheum Dis 72(6):858–862

Chapter 2
Pharmacotherapy of Rheumatoid Arthritis

Aygin Bayraktar-Ekincioglu and Louise Grech

2.1 Introduction

Panacea, or Panakeia, was the Greek goddess of healing and was attributed to have a potion that cures all illnesses and diseases. Being the daughter of Asclepius, son of Apollo and god of medicine, she was venerated in the temple dedicated to Asclepius, in Epidaurus in the northeast of the beautiful Peloponnese. She is also mentioned in the original Hippocratic oath where the physician swears by a number of gods to serve the patients to the best of one's abilities. Although the quest for a universal cure, an elixir of life, or the holy grail of medicine remains a mythological fictional aspect, medicine has made great progress when it comes to the drug armamentarium available for rheumatoid arthritis. This chapter puts forward the pharmacological management of rheumatoid arthritis starting with a look at the past.

2.2 From Peruvian Bark to Biologic Era

The possible first documented use of effective drugs in the management of rheumatoid arthritis dates to 1680 when physicians administered Peruvian bark containing the antimalarial agent, quinine, whose properties were first found to be effective for

A. Bayraktar-Ekincioglu, PhD (✉)
Department of Clinical Pharmacy, Faculty of Pharmacy, Hacettepe University,
Ankara, Turkey
e-mail: aygin@hacettepe.edu.tr

L. Grech, PhD (✉)
Clinical Pharmacy Practice Unit, Department of Pharmacy, Mater Dei Hospital,
Msida, Malta

Department of Pharmacy, Faculty of Medicine and Surgery, University of Malta, Msida, Malta
e-mail: louise.grech@um.edu.mt

© Springer Science+Business Media Singapore 2016
L. Grech, A. Lau (eds.), *Pharmaceutical Care Issues of Patients
with Rheumatoid Arthritis*, DOI 10.1007/978-981-10-1421-5_2

management of systemic lupus erythematosus [1]. Between 1897 and 1899, Dr Felix Hoffmann and the pharmaceutical company Bayer synthesised chemically, manufactured, and patented aspirin as a drug (acetylsalicylic acid derived from willow bark) which, due to its anti-inflammatory effects, was used in the treatment of rheumatoid arthritis [2]. In 1929, administration of parenteral gold or sodium aurothiomalate was introduced to alleviate pain in rheumatoid arthritis paving the way for a new class of drugs later to be called disease-modifying antirheumatic drugs (DMARDs) [3]. Subsequently in the 1940s, Professor Svartz from Sweden in collaboration with the manufacturing company Pharmacia developed sulfasalazine [4, 5], and in 1949, Philip Hench from Mayo Clinic presented a paper on the use of cortisone in the treatment of rheumatoid arthritis during the 7th International Congress of Rheumatology in New York [6]. Hench and colleagues were awarded the Nobel Prize for Medicine in 1950 for their contribution to furthering the knowledge on rheumatoid arthritis. In the 1970s, studies carried out using penicillamine in rheumatoid arthritis showed that this product was effective in 60% of the patients but had a high toxicity profile, including rash, stomatitis, metallic taste, proteinuria and myelosuppression. Lack of evidence that penicillamine decreases radiological progression of the disease led to a gradual decrease in the use of penicillamine as a disease-modifying antirheumatic drug [7, 8]. A major breakthrough came in the 1980s when methotrexate was introduced in the treatment of rheumatoid arthritis. Ironically, methotrexate was first studied at low doses in the treatment of rheumatoid arthritis in the 1960s; however, due to concerns about its safety, being a cytotoxic drug, methotrexate was not very much used in the 1960s. It was only later on in the 1980s that several studies confirmed the efficacy and safety of methotrexate in rheumatoid arthritis, and thereafter, methotrexate gained its position as the "gold standard" and one of the most effective DMARDs [9–12]. In 1987, leflunomide was shown to be effective in rheumatoid arthritis in rats, and later on, its clinical efficacy and safety was demonstrated in humans [13, 14].

The 1990s exposed another breakthrough in the management of rheumatoid arthritis through the identification and implication of the pro-inflammatory markers such as tumour necrosis factor alpha (TNFα) and interleukin-1(IL-1) and interleukin-6 (IL-6). This was the start of the biologic era which led to the marketing and successful administration of tumour necrosis factor inhibitors such as etanercept, infliximab, adalimumab, golimumab and certolizumab, the B-cell blocker rituximab, the interleukin-1 receptor antagonist anakinra and the interleukin-6 receptor blocker tocilizumab [15–20]. The biologic era revolutionised the pharmacotherapeutic pyramidal approach in rheumatoid arthritis.

2.3   Treatment Shift: The Inverted Pyramidal Approach

In rheumatoid arthritis, health care providers aim to:

1. Provide symptom relief, namely, eliminate or decrease pain, stiffness and swelling
2. Slow and, if possible, arrest disease progression in order to preserve functionality by maintaining joint stability and mobility and prevent structural damage to the joints

3. Prevent and manage extra-articular complications and co-morbidities particularly, preserve/protect cardiovascular profile and prevent opportunistic infections
4. Educate patients and their carers and keep them central to decision-making
5. Maintain and possibly improve the patients' quality of life

Drug therapy for rheumatoid arthritis is directed at achieving these five aims. The overarching principle is to "treat to target" as early as possible to arrest the disease progression and aim for remission [21–25]. As discussed in Chap. 1, early diagnosis and appropriate management of rheumatoid arthritis have become an important factor which dictates prognosis and possible remission [26–31]. Against such a background, the availability, specificity, efficacy and safety of biological monoclonal antibodies which target specific pro-inflammatory cytokines such as tumour necrosis factor alpha, interleukin-6 and CD20 B-cells have changed considerably the pharmacotherapy of rheumatoid arthritis and led to the inverted pyramidal approach.

Initially, the pyramidal approach and treatment guidelines were based on initiating treatment through symptom relief drugs followed by gradual intensified anti-inflammatory agents. Essentially, analgesics were therefore used as first-line drugs. If the symptoms of rheumatoid arthritis remained uncontrolled, or if there was radiological evidence of disease progression, a second-line drug would be considered. The disease-modifying antirheumatic drugs (DMARDs) such as methotrexate, sulfasalazine and leflunomide were the mainstay second-line agents in treatment. In the event that the selected disease-modifying drug was not effective, sequential and, or, combination therapy using more than one DMARD would be considered. Corticosteroids were considered as third-line agents [32–34]. At this stage, the treatment strategy was to preserve the most effective (and less well tolerated) DMARDs until disease progression dictated a *move up* the pyramid. This "move up" trend within the pyramid was based on the assumptions that rheumatoid arthritis is a benign non-life-threatening disease, aspirin and non-steroidal anti-inflammatory drug therapy are mild therapeutic options and DMARDs are too toxic for routine use [35]. Clinically, this pyramidal approach meant that the patients were being offered primarily symptom relief, but very little was being done to prevent disease progression, decrease joint destruction and improve long-term outcomes.

The awareness that rheumatoid arthritis causes substantial morbidity and mortality and is not a benign disease as well as the understanding that, if appropriately used through regular monitoring, DMARDs are no more toxic than non-steroidal anti-inflammatory drugs but are more effective in reducing the radiological progression of the disease, led to an updated pyramidal approach: the inverted pyramidal approach [36–45].

The importance of early referral of rheumatoid arthritis patients by general practitioners to rheumatologists became a focal issue in the use of disease-modifying antirheumatic drugs earlier on during the course of rheumatoid arthritis [46–48]. In 2002, treatment recommendations issued by the American College of Rheumatology (ACR), stipulated that all patients with rheumatoid arthritis were eligible for administration of DMARDs and this should not be delayed beyond 3 months from the time of diagnosis of rheumatoid arthritis [49]. At this stage, pharmacological management relied on the prescribing of DMARDs as first-line therapy, while analgesics were used on a "prn" or as required basis to control pain and achieve pain free state in patients' daily life.

Between 2008 and 2015 the traditional pyramidal approach was updated by newer treatment guidelines issued by both the American College of Rheumatology and the European League Against Rheumatism (EULAR) [50–54]. Although both entities have their own separate evidenced-based guidelines, the respective recommendations mirror each other and essentially advocate the rapid move to the use of highly effective biological agents to achieve a clinical remission state of rheumatoid arthritis. Figure 2.1 schematically illustrates the shift in the pharmacotherapeutic management of rheumatoid arthritis over time.

2.4   Disease-Modifying Antirheumatic Drugs: Synthetic and Biologic DMARDs

Disease-modifying antirheumatic drugs (DMARDs) are immunosuppressant drugs which target progression of rheumatoid arthritis. The development and use of biologic drugs within the drug armamentarium led to further classification and clarification in the nomenclature used when referring to DMARDs as a class of drugs used in rheumatology, similar to the way in which NSAIDs refer to the class of non-steroidal anti-inflammatory drugs. DMARDs can be subdivided into synthetic DMARDs (sDMARDs) or biologic DMARDs (bDMARDs) [55].

Synthetic DMARDS (sDMARDs), as the name implies, are synthetic and chemical in nature. They commonly have a slow onset of action (at least 12 weeks or 3 months) and their mode of action is not fully understood. Synthetic DMARDs can be used as monotherapy or in a combination with steroids or other DMARDs They are all relatively cheap and most are administered via the oral route. Examples include methotrexate, sulfasalazine, hydroxychloroquine, leflunomide and the newer janus kinase inhibitor, tofacitinib.

In contrast, *biologic* DMARDS are biologic medicinal products having a relatively fast onset of action resulting in patients immediately reporting some benefit following initiation of therapy. Their effectiveness stems from the specificity to target precise pro-inflammatory markers within the inflammatory cascade. Being biologic in nature, there is an element of immunogenicity as well as issues on biosimilarity and being protein in nature, their stability is highly effected by warm temperatures. Biologic drugs are more expensive than synthetic DMARDs.

The advent of biosimilars has introduced a certain degree of competitiveness with respect to pricing but the decline in the prices leaves much to be desired and the biologic originators and biosimilars are still relatively expensive compared to synthetic DMARDs. The launch of biosimilars has also added a further complexity in the nomenclature of DMARDs. In 2014, Smolen et al, proposed a nomenclature system to distinguish between originator and biosimilar products. The proposed system recommends *boDMARDs* as biologic originator products versus *bsDMARDs* which refers to biosimilar DMARDs [55].

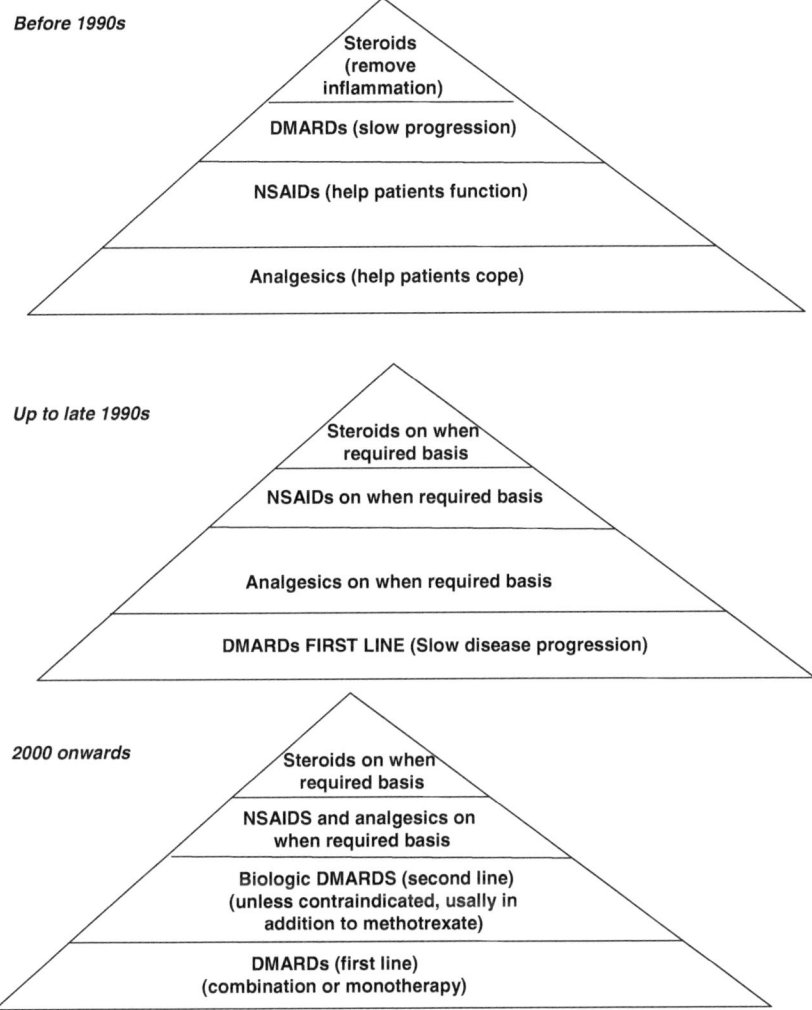

Fig. 2.1 Transformation of the pyramid pharmacological approach (Source: Adapted and updated from: Azzopardi [108])

2.5   Synthetic DMARDs

The efficacy of synthetic DMARDs in the management of rheumatoid arthritis has stood the test of time and these drugs are considered essential in the management of the condition [56, 57]. They are the first-line drugs recommended by clinical guidelines. In the following section an overview of the most commonly used synthetic DMARDs is given.

2.5.1 Methotrexate: Not Just a Chemotherapy Drug

Methotrexate is a commonly used first-line synthetic DMARD as evidenced by the latest clinical guidelines and literature reviews [53, 54, 56–60]. Methotrexate is a folate antagonist which acts by inhibiting the enzyme dihydrofolate reductase (DHFR). Dihydrofolate reductase catalyses the reduction of dihydrofolate to tetrahydrofolate (FH_4) thereby blocking the regeneration of FH_4 and preventing the synthesis of purines and pyrimidines which are essential for DNA and RNA synthesis. Methotrexate inhibits the metabolism of actively dividing cells such as those involved in the inflammatory immune cascade within rheumatoid arthritis [61].

2.5.1.1 Dosage and Administration

In rheumatoid arthritis the initial dose is usually 7.5 mg once a week taken orally on the same day each week. The maximum dosage is 25 mg once a week [62, 63]. In general, the prescribed dose is administered as a single weekly dose. However, in order to reduce the incidence of gastrointestinal side effects such as nausea, diarrhoea and vomiting patients prone to such side effects can be advised to take the prescribed dose in divided doses taken over a 24-h period [64]. Methotrexate is usually administered as oral preparation in the form of tablets. Parenteral preparations of methotrexate administered as intramuscular or subcutaneous preparations offer the advantage of having less incidence of gastrointestinal side effects and greater efficacy secondary to higher dose and better bioavailability when compared to the oral route [65–69].

2.5.1.2 Contraindications to Methotrexate Therapy

Methotrexate is metabolised by the liver and excreted in urine. Patients with renal impairment will show decreased overall methotrexate clearance and dose adjustments are recommended in patients with renal impairment and methotrexate should be completely avoided in severe renal impairment. Methotrexate is not dialysed and therefore is contraindicated in patients with haemodialysis or continuous ambulatory peritoneal dialysis. It is also contraindicated in chronic liver impairment. Concurrent intake of alcohol tends to contribute to liver damage and hence excessive alcohol ingestion is contraindicated. Methotrexate is also contraindicated in the presence of pre-existing pulmonary disease, severe and serious infections, immunodeficiency states and bone marrow suppression such as blood dyscrasias [62, 63].

2.5.1.3 Side Effects of Methotrexate

Gastrointestinal side effects such as nausea, vomiting, oral ulceration, minor hair thinning, abdominal discomfort, diarrhoea and headache are the most common side effects of methotrexate. Bone marrow suppression, acute pneumonitis or chronic pulmonary fibrosis as well as liver or renal toxicity are also part of the side effect profile of methotrexate [62, 63]. Liver toxicity generally presents itself by an elevated level of transaminases liver function tests.

The co-administration of folic acid may reduce the possibility of nausea, anorexia, oral ulceration, abdominal discomfort and diarrhoea as well as the incidence of bone marrow suppression [70–72].

2.5.2 Sulfasalazine

Sulfasalazine was developed in the 1940s as a synthetic disease-modifying antirheumatic drug and remains highly prescribed because of its low toxicity profile and its high efficacy. Sulfasalazine is essentially a prodrug which is metabolised to the active sulfapyridine and 5-aminosalicylic acid. Patients allergic to sulfa components cannot be administered sulfasalazine. Its mode of action remains largely unclear but it offers anti-inflammatory and immunomodulatory properties [60, 73].

2.5.2.1 Dosage and Administration

Sulfasalazine is prescribed orally at an initial dose of 500 mg daily which can be increased by increments of 500 mg to a maximum dose of 3 g daily in divided doses [62, 63].

2.5.2.2 Contraindications to Sulfasalazine

Sulfasalazine is contraindicated in patients allergic to sulfa drugs and patients suffering from porphyria, intestinal and urinary obstruction, and used with caution in patients with renal or hepatic impairment and severe asthma [62, 63].

2.5.2.3 Side Effects of Sulfasalazine

Sulfasalazine is generally well tolerated. Common side effects include nausea, diarrhoea, headache, and oral ulcerations. Rash, reversible oligospermia, abnormal liver and renal function and bone marrow suppression may occur [62, 63]. Patients suffering from glucose-6-phosphatedehydrogenase (G6PD) deficiency are at an increased risk of developing haemolytic anaemia [60]. Sulfasalazine is excreted in most body fluids including urine and this may lead to yellow discolouration of the urine as well as staining of soft coloured lenses [62, 63].

Sulfasalazine tends to inhibit the absorption of folic acid and may cause folate deficiency. In such cases, folic acid supplementation may be necessary [60].

2.5.3   Leflunomide

Leflunomide is a modern synthetic disease-modifying antirheumatic drug having both immunomodulatory and anti-inflammatory properties. Leflunomide is an isoxazole derivative which is activated through hepatic metabolism. The active metabolite, teriflunomide, binds to dihydro-orotate dehydrogenase and acts by inhibiting the synthesis of pyrimidine nucleotides in immune cells, particularly the T cells thereby reducing the pro-cytokines-tumour necrosis factor (TNF) and interleukin 1 (11-1) [60, 73, 74]. Leflunomide has a long half-life of approximately 2 weeks [62, 63, 75].

2.5.3.1   Dosage and Administration

Leflunomide is administered as a loading dose of 100 mg daily for the first 3 days and thereafter at a maintenance dose of 10–20 mg daily. Omitting the loading dose and starting immediately at a dose of 20 mg daily tends to result in less incidence of side effects and less discontinuation rates [62, 63, 76].

2.5.3.2   Contraindications to Leflunomide

Leflunomide is contraindicated in patients with liver and renal impairment including conditions where there is hypoproteinaemia. It is also contraindicated in patients with severe and serious infections, immunodeficiency states and bone marrow suppression [62, 63].

2.5.3.3   Side Effects of Leflunomide

Leflunomide is generally well tolerated. The most common side effects are gastrointestinal discomfort, reversible alopecia, rash and particularly hypertension. Liver function may also be affected resulting in abnormal liver function tests [62, 63]. A washout procedure is required to eliminate the drug from the body prior to starting another disease-modifying antirheumatic drug, in the presence of a serious side effect or prior to conception. In this case, leflunomide therapy should be stopped and cholestyramine 8 g three times daily or activated charcoal 50 g four times daily are administered for 11 days. The concentration of the active metabolite should be less than 20 µg/l measured on two occasions 14 days apart [63].

2.5.4   Hydroxychloroquine

Hydroxychloroquine and chloroquine are antimalarial drugs which exert their immunosuppressive effect through the suppression of lysosomal enzymes. Pro-inflammatory cytokines are implicated in the inflammatory response related to rheumatoid arthritis [77–79].

2.5.4.1   Dosage and Administration

Hydroxychloroquine is prescribed at a dose of 400 mg in divided doses [62, 63].

2.5.4.2   Contraindications to Hydroxychloroquine

Hydroxychloroquine is contraindicated in patients who are allergic to 4-aminoquinoline derivatives, suffering from retinal problems, porphyria, psoriasis, severe renal and liver impairment [62, 63].

2.5.4.3   Side Effects of Hydroxychloroquine

The most common side effects are due to gastrointestinal toxicity. The serious side effect is retinal damage occurring as hydroxychloroquine accumulates in the melanotic retinal pigment epithelium gradually damaging the retinal pigment, epithelium and the retina. Retinal toxicity is more likely to occur in association with doses greater than 400 mg and in patients older than 70 years [62, 63]. Other side effects include blurred vision, accommodation difficulty, headache, rashes, abnormal skin pigmentation and pruritus, ECG changes, convulsions, keratopathy, ototoxicity and hair loss. Neuropathy, myopathy and bone marrow suppression may also occur [62, 63].

2.5.5   Other Less Commonly Used Synthetic DMARDs

Azathioprine is an oral purine analogue thought to exert its immunosuppressive action by the inhibition of lymphocyte proliferation [73]. Nausea, vomiting and diarrhoea are commonly occurring side effects which tend to occur early on during treatment. Bone marrow suppression and liver toxicity may also occur. Azathioprine is administered initially at a dose of 1 mg/kg/day increasing to a maximum of 2.5 mg/kg/day [62, 63].

Ciclosporin is another immunosuppressive agent which is mainly used for the prevention of organ rejection in transplantation. In 1994, ciclosporin was licensed for treatment of rheumatoid arthritis [80]. Ciclosporin inhibits T-lymphocyte and lymphokine production which are implicated in inflammation associated with the pathogenesis of rheumatoid arthritis. Common side effects include paraesthesia, tremor, headaches, hypertrichosis, gingival hypertrophy, hirsutism, nausea, hypertension, renal impairment and bone marrow suppression. It is prescribed at a dose of 2.5 mg/kg/day in 2 divided doses and increased to a maximum of 4.5 mg/kg/day, according to tolerance [62, 63].

Parenteral sodium aurothiomalate or gold, is another effective synthetic DMARD indicated in rheumatoid arthritis. Common side effects include rashes, stomatitis, bone marrow suppression and proteinuria. Long-term use of gold injection may lead to greyish blue discolouration of the skin which may be confused with cyanosis [62, 63].

2.6   Biologic DMARDs: Latest Treatment Modalities

Biologic DMARDs target specific pro-inflammatory cytokines implicated in the inflammatory cascade of rheumatoid arthritis. Table 2.1 gives an overview of the currently available biologic DMARDs used in rheumatoid arthritis.

Table 2.1 Biologic DMARDS licensed in rheumatoid arthritis

Biologic DMARD	Class	Dose	Licensing
Adalimumab	TNF inhibitor (recombinant human monoclonal antibody)	40 mg every fortnight to 40 mg every week administered subcutaneously	As monotherapy or with methotrexate
Certolizumab	TNF inhibitor (recombinant humanised monoclonal antibody)	Administered subcutaneously Loading dose of 400 mg at week 0, 2, 4 Maintenance dose of 200 mg every 2 weeks or 400 mg every 4 weeks	As monotherapy or with methotrexate
Etanercept	TNF inhibitor (fusion protein receptor)	50 mg every week administered subcutaneously	As monotherapy or with methotrexate
Golimumab	TNF inhibitor (recombinant human monoclonal antibody)	50 mg once a month administered subcutaneously	In combination with methotrexate
Infliximab	TNF inhibitor (chimeric monoclonal antibody)	Administered as intravenous infusion Loading dose: 3 mg/kg at week 0, 2, 6 (given over 2 h) Maintenance dose: 3 mg/kg every 8 weeks increased to a maximum of 3 mg/kg every 4 weeks or 7.5 mg/kg every 8 weeks Maintenance dose can be given over 1 h provided the patient never had infusion reactions and the dose does not exceed 6 mg/kg Pre-medication with antihistamine + paracetamol + steroid combination can be considered	In combination with methotrexate Infliximab is licensed with methotrexate in order to reduce the risk of developing auto-antibody against infliximab and increase tolerance during treatment
Anakinra	Interleukin-1 antagonist (recombinant *E. coli*-derived monoclonal antibody)	100 mg daily administered subcutaneously	In combination with methotrexate

(continued)

Table 2.1 (continued)

Biologic DMARD	Class	Dose	Licensing
Tocilizumab	Interleukin 6 antagonist (recombinant humanised monoclonal antibody)	Administered as 162 mg subcutaneously every week *OR* Administered over 1 h intravenously at a dose of 8 mg/kg with a maximum dose of 800 mg every 4 weeks	As monotherapy or with methotrexate
Abatacept	T-lymphocyte inhibitor (chimeric fusion protein)	Administered as 125 mg subcutaneously every week *OR* As intravenous infusion over 30 min with a loading dose at week 0, 2, 4 and maintenance every 4 weeks. The dose is weight dependent. Patients weighing less than 60 kg are administered 500 mg each time. Patients weighing between 60 and 100 kg are given a dose of 750 mg. Patients weighing more than 100 kg are administered a dose of 1 g each time	In combination with methotrexate
Rituximab	Anti-CD20 antigen (chimeric monoclonal antibody)	Administered as 1 g day 1 and day 15 Premedications are always required	In combination with methotrexate

All biologic DMARDs present similar side effect profiles, contraindications and cautions. In general, all biologic drugs are potent immunosuppressors and are associated with an increased risk for infections. In view of this, all patients who are to be prescribed a biologic DMARD should be pre-screened to eliminate the possibility of serious infections such as tuberculosis, hepatitis B, hepatitis C and Human Immunodeficiency Virus (HIV). Live vaccines are contraindicated are in all patients on biologic DMARDs since the patients will not be able to mount a full immune response and the risk of actually getting the full blown infection from the live component of the vaccine is high [49–54, 56, 81–85].

Anakinra (interleukin-1 antagonist) and abatacept (T-lymphocyte blocker) are implicated in causing severe infections in patients suffering with asthma or chronic obstructive pulmonary disease, respectively. Therefore they are to be used with caution in these patients [81–85].

Tumour necrosis factor inhibitors are contraindicated in patients with severe congestive heart failure as they can cause worsening of the congestive heart failure. Tumour necrosis factor inhibitors can also cause demyelination and are therefore contraindicated in multiple sclerosis and demyelinating disease. Etanercept and infliximab have been implicated in causing lupus-like syndrome [49–54, 56, 81–85].

The Interleukin-6 receptor antagonist, tocilizumab has been associated with gastrointestinal perforations in patients with inflammatory bowel disease and is therefore avoided in these patients. It is also associated with a higher incidence of elevated transaminases and lipid profile when compared to other biologic drugs which do not report such side effects [85, 86].

Rituximab, is associated with a higher incidence of the rare progressive multifocal leucoencephalopathy [85, 92]. It is interesting to note that rituximab is not licensed as monotherapy but the 2011 British Society for Rheumatology (BSR), British Health Professionals in Rheumatology (BHPR) guidelines recommend its use with leflunomide or as monotherapy when methotrexate is contraindicated [93].

The higher risk of malignancy associated with biologic drugs, is debatable as to whether the risk is associated with the drugs themselves or with the continuous inflammation secondary to the condition itself. Nevertheless, clinically, biologic drugs are contraindicated in patients with active malignancy with the exception of rituximab which may be part of chemotherapy [87–92].

2.7   Treatment Strategies

In summary, in accordance with the latest guidelines separately put forward by the European League against Rheumatism and the American College of Rheumatology, the first-line treatment in rheumatoid arthritis remains the use of synthetic DMARDs, specifically methotrexate [53, 54]. The choice of the first-line synthetic DMARD is based on the efficacy, side effect profile, monitoring requirements, convenience of administration and cost of the medication. Methotrexate is the ideal candidate offering efficacy combined with low toxicity profile, convenient administration and a good price. It is considered to be the gold standard synthetic DMARD. Sulfasalazine and leflunomide are equally effective to methotrexate offering a comparable low toxicity profile which is why guidelines recommend their use in case of methotrexate intolerance or in cases where methotrexate is contraindicated [53, 54, 94–97]. Parenteral sodium aurothiomalate is equally effective but its side effect profile together with the need for urinalysis prior to each dose administration has limited its use and hence sodium aurothiomalate is no longer commonly used in rheumatoid arthritis [98]. Hydroxychloroquine is a synthetic DMARD with a limited role in mild to moderate rheumatoid arthritis. It is however the mainstay therapy in systemic lupus erythematosus [99].

The use of combination synthetic DMARDs is considered as second line therapy when there is failure to achieve a good response with a first single-agent synthetic DMARD within 6 months of initiation of therapy. However, in the presence of poor prognostic factors such as early joint erosion, high ESR and anti-CCP, there is an overall preference to rapidly move to the addition of a biologic DMARD rather than a combination of synthetic DMARDs [53, 54]. In general, tumour necrosis factor inhibitors are recommended as the first biologic DMARDs to be prescribed followed by a choice of the other classes of biologic DMARDs. In cases where patients remain uncontrolled despite the administration of a synthetic DMARD and a biologic DMARD, the biologic DMARD can be changed. It is important to note however that a combination of biologic DMARDs is strongly not recommended due to the increased risk of immunosuppression [53, 54].

2.7.1 Treatment Strategies in Pregnancy and Breastfeeding: What Are the Options?

As already stated in Chap. 1, unlike systemic lupus erythematosus, rheumatoid arthritis tends to calm down during pregnancy which puts the clinician's mind at rest since most of the DMARDs are contraindicated in pregnancy and breastfeeding. Methotrexate is teratogenic and is therefore contraindicated in pregnancy. Male patients should wait a minimum period of 3 months after discontinuation of therapy whereas females must wait at least one ovulatory cycle after discontinuation of methotrexate therapy before considering pregnancy. The same goes for leflunomide which is also contraindicated in pregnancy and breastfeeding [100–106].

Sulfasalazine, hydroxychloroquine, azathioprine and ciclosporin are recommended as safe to administer during pregnancy and breastfeeding even though the respective summary of product characteristics advice avoidance of the respective drugs during pregnancy and breastfeeding [100–106].

There is debatable evidence with respect to the use of biologics in pregnancy and breastfeeding. The official guidelines on their use in pregnancy and breastfeeding were only recently put forward by the British Society for Rheumatology [106]. Soon after, the EULAR issued similar suggestions to aid clinicians during decision-making when it comes to the use of biologics in pregnancy and breastfeeding [107]. The guidelines recommend that infliximab can be continued until 16 weeks of pregnancy. Etanercept and adalimumab can be used until the end of the second semester whereas certolizumab can be continued till the end of the pregnancy. No data is put forward for golimumab. Breastfeeding is recommended with caution in female patients on tumour necrosis factor inhibitors. The guidelines strictly recommend that rituximab should be stopped 6 months prior to conception whereas tocilizumab should be stopped 3 months prior to conception. Both are not compatible with breastfeeding. There is lack of data with respect to abatacept and anakinra which is why these are recommended as contraindicated in pregnancy and breastfeeding [106].

Take Home Messages
- The introduction of biologic DMARDs has revolutionised the pharmacotherapy of rheumatoid arthritis.
- Latest guidelines put forward by the EULAR and the ACR recommend the use of methotrexate as first-line synthetic DMARD.
- Biologic DMARDs are recommended in patients who have failed to achieve a clinical response with methotrexate monotherapy or methotrexate in addition to other synthetic DMARDs.
- Biologic DMARDs are potent immunosuppressants and cannot be prescribed together, in combination.
- Methotrexate and leflunomide are contraindicated in pregnancy and breastfeeding.
- The British Society for Rheumatology have issued guidelines on the use of biologic drugs during pregnancy and breastfeeding to guide clinicians in decision-making.

References

1. Canavese P, Fogell RW (2008) Arthritis: changes in its prevalence during the nineteenth and twentieth centuries. In: Cutler DM, Wise DA (eds) Health at older ages: the causes and consequences of declining disability among the elderly. The University of Chicago Press, Chicago, p 56
2. Connelly D. A history of Aspirin. Clin Pharm. 2014;6(7). doi:10.1211/CP.2014.20066661
3. Forestier J (1935) Rheumatoid arthritis and its treatment with gold salts – a result of six years experience. J Lab Clin Med 20:827–840
4. Box SA, Pullar T (1997) Sulfasalazine in the treatment of rheumatoid arthritis. Br J Rheumatol 36:382–386
5. Snaeder W (2005) Drug discovery. Wiley, Chichester, p 398
6. Glyn JH (1998) The discovery of cortisone – a personal memory. Brit Med J 317:822
7. Multicentre Trial Group (1973) Controlled trial of D-penicillamine in rheumatoid arthritis. Lancet 1:275–285
8. Dixon ASJ, Davies J, Dormandy TL, Hamilton EB, Holt PJ, Mason RM et al (1975) Synthetic D-penicillamine in rheumatoid arthritis. Double blind controlled study of a high and low dosage regimen. Ann Rheum Dis 34:416–421
9. Ward JR (1985) Historical perspective on the use of Methotrexate for the treatment of rheumatoid arthritis. J Rheumatol 12(Suppl 12):3–6
10. Weinblatt ME, Coblyn JS, Fox DA, Fraser PA, Holdsworth DE, Glass DN et al (1985) Efficacy of low dose methotrexate in rheumatoid arthritis. New Engl J Med 312(13):818–822
11. Weinblatt ME, Weissman BN, Holdsworth DE, Fraser PA, Maier AL, Falchuk KR (1992) Long-term prospective study of methotrexate in the treatment of rheumatoid arthritis. 84-month update. Arthritis Rheum 35(2):129–137
12. Weinblatt ME (2013) Methetrexate in rheumatoid arthritis: a quarter century of development. Trans Am Clin Climatol Assoc 124:16–25
13. Pasternak RD, Wadopain NS, Wright RN, Siminoff P, Gylys JA, Buyniski JP (1987) Disease modifying activity of HWA 486 (leflunomide) in rat adjuvant-induced arthritis. Agents Actions 21(3–4):241–243
14. Kalden JR, Schattenkirchner M, Sorensen H, Emery P, Deighton C, Rozman B et al (2003) The efficacy and safety of leflunomide in patients with active rheumatoid arthritis: a 5 year follow up study. Ann Rheum Dis 48(6):1513–1520
15. Kalden JR, Manger B (1995) Biologic agents in the treatment of inflammatory rheumatic diseases. Curr Opin Rheumatol 7(3):191–197
16. Strand V (1998) Future use of biologic agents alone or in combination for the treatment of rheumatoid arthritis. Z Rheumatol 57(1):41–45
17. Furst DE, Breedveld FC, Kalden JR, Smolen JS, Burmester GR, Dougados M et al (2003) Updated consensus statement on biological agents for the treatment of rheumatoid arthritis and other immune mediated inflammatory diseases (May 2003). Ann Rheum Dis 62(Suppl 2):2–9
18. Scott DL, Kingsley GH. Biologics in rheumatoid arthritis. In: Scott DL, Kingsley GH, editors (2008) Inflammatory arthritis in clinical practice. London, Springer; pp 86–89
19. Curtis JR, Singh JA (2011) Use of biologics in rheumatoid arthritis: current and emerging paradigms of care. Clin Ther 33(6):679–707
20. Malviya G, Salemi S, Lagana B, Diamanti AP, D'Amelio R, Signore A (2013) Biological therapies for rheumatoid arthritis: progress to date. BioDrugs 27(4):329–345
21. Emery P, Salmon M (1995) Early rheumatoid arthritis: time to aim for remission? Ann Rheum Dis 54:944–947
22. Smolen JS, Aletaha D (2006) What should be our treatment goal in rheumatoid arthritis today? Clin Exp Rheumatol 24(Suppl 43):S7–S13
23. Smolen JS, Aletaha D, Bijlsma JWJ, Breedveld FC, Boumpas D, Burmester G et al (2010) Treating rheumatoid arthritis to target: recommendations of an international task force. Ann Rheum Dis 69:631–637

24. Schoels M, Knevel R, Aletaha D, Bijlsma JW, Breedveld FC, Boumpas DT et al (2010) Evidence for treating rheumatoid arthritis to target: results of a systematic literature search. Ann Rheum Dis 69:638–643
25. Smolen JS, Breedveld FC, Burmester G, Bykerk V, Dougados M, Emery P et al (2015) Treating rheumatoid arthritis to target: 2014 update of the recommendations of an international task force. Ann Rheum Dis 75:3–15. doi:10.1136/annrheumdis-2015.207524
26. Finckh A, Liang MH, van Herckenrode CM, de Pablo P (2006) Long term impact of early treatment on radiographic progression in rheumatoid arthritis: a meta-analysis. Arthritis Care Res 55(6):864–872
27. Combe B, Landewe R, Lukas C (2007) EULAR recommendations for the management of early arthritis: report of a task force of the European Standing Committee for International Clinical Studies Including Therapeutics (ESCISIT). Ann Rheum Dis 66:34–45
28. Klarenbeek NB, van der Kooiji SM, Guler-Yuksel M, van Groenendael JHLM, Han KH, Kerstens PJSM et al (2011) Discontinuing treatment in patients with rheumatoid arthritis in sustained clinical remission: exploratory analyses from the BeSt study. Ann Rheum Dis 70(2):315–319
29. Kyburz D, Gabay C, Michel BA, Finckh A (2011) The long-term impact of early treatment of rheumatoid arthritis on radiographic progression: a population based cohort study. Rheumatology 50(6):1106–1110
30. Schneider M, Kruger K (2013) Rheumatoid arthritis – early diagnosis and disease management. Dtsch Arztebl Int 110(27–28):477–484
31. Raza K, Filer A (2015) The therapeutic window of opportunity in rheumatoid arthritis: does it ever close? Ann Rheum Dis 74(5):793–794
32. Platt P (1997) Rheumatoid arthritis and its treatment. Pharm J 259:298–301
33. Parkinson S, Alldred A (2002) Drug regimens for rheumatoid arthritis. Hospital Pharm 9:11–15
34. Choy EH (2004) Two is better than one? Combination therapy in rheumatoid arthritis. Rheumatology 43(10):1205–1207
35. Scott DL, Shipley M, Dawson A, Edwards S, Symmons DPM, Woolf AD (1998) The clinical management of rheumatoid arthritis and osteoarthritis: strategies for improving clinical effectiveness. Br J Rheumatol 37:546–554
36. Fries JF, Williams CA, Bloch DA (1993) The relative toxicity of disease modifying anti-rheumatic drugs. Arthritis Rheum 36:297–306
37. Fries JF, Williams CA, Morfeld D, Singh G, Sibley J (1996) Reduction in long term disability in patients with rheumatoid arthritis by disease modifying anti-rheumatic drug based treatment strategies. Arthritis Rheum 39:616–622
38. van der Heide A, Jacobs JWG, Bijlsma JWJ, Heurkens AHM, van Booma-Frankfort C, van der Veen MJ, Haanen HCB, Hofman DM (1996) The effectiveness of early treatment with second line anti-rheumatic drugs. Ann Intern Med 124:699–707
39. Wollheim FA (1997) Disease modifying drugs in rheumatoid arthritis. BMJ 314:766
40. Abu-Shakra M, Toker R, Flusser D, Flusser G, Friger M, Sukenik S et al (1998) Clinical and radiographic outcomes of rheumatoid arthritis patients not treated with disease modifying drugs. Arthritis Rheum 41:1190–1195
41. Irvine S, Munro R, Porter D (1999) Early referral, diagnosis and treatment of rheumatoid arthritis: evidence for changing medical practice. Ann Rheum Dis 58:510–513
42. Fries JF (2000) Current treatment paradigms in rheumatoid arthritis. Rheumatology 39(Suppl 1):30–35
43. Pincus T, Ferraccioli G, Sokka T, Larsen A, Rau R, Kushner I, Wolfe F (2002) Evidence from clinical trials and long-term observational studies that disease modifying rheumatic drugs slow radiographic progression in rheumatoid arthritis: updating a 1983 review. Rheumatology 41:1346–1356
44. Upchurch KS, Kay J (2012) Evolution of the treatment for rheumatoid arthritis. Rheumatology 51(Suppl 6):vi28–vi36
45. Smolen JS, Aletaha D (2015) Rheumatoid arthritis therapy reappraisal: strategies, opportunities, challenges. Nat Rev Rheumatol 11:276–289

46. Emery P, Breedveld FC, Dougados M, Kalden JR, Schiff MH, Smolen JS (2002) Early referral recommendation for newly diagnosed rheumatoid arthritis: evidence-based development of a clinical guide. Ann Rheum Dis 61:290–297
47. Villeneuve E, Nam JL, Bell MJ, Deighton CM, Felson DT, Hazes JM et al (2013) A systematic literature review of strategies promoting early referral and reducing delays in the diagnosis and management of inflammatory arthritis. Ann Rheum Dis 72:13–22
48. Cummins LL, Vangaveti V, Roberts JL (2015) Rheumatoid arthritis referrals and rheumatologists scarcity: a prioritization tool. Arthritis Care Res 67(3):326–331
49. American College of Rheumatology Subcomittee on Rheumatoid Arthritis Guidelines (2002) Guidelines for management of rheumatoid arthritis 2002 update. Arthritis Rheum 46:328–346
50. Saag KG, Teng GG, Patkar NM, Anuntiyo J, Finney C, Curtis JR et al (2008) American College of Rheumatology 2008 recommendations for the use of nonbiologic and biologic disease modifying antirheumatic drugs in rheumatoid arthritis. Arthritis Rheum 59:762–784
51. Smolen JS, Landewe R, Breedveld FC et al (2010) EULAR recommendations for the management of rheumatoid arthritis with synthetic and biological disease-modifying antirheumatic drugs. Ann Rheum Dis 69:964–975
52. Singh JA, Furst DE, Bharat A, Curtis JF, Kavanaugh AF, Kremer JM et al (2012) 2012 update of the 2008 American College of Rheumatology recommendations for the use of disease-modifying antirheumatic drugs and biologic agents in the treatment of rheumatoid arthritis. Arthritis Care Res 64(5):625–639
53. Smolen JS, Landewe R, Breedveld FC, Buch M, Burmester G, Dougados M et al (2014) EULAR recommendations for the management of rheumatoid arthritis with synthetic and biological disease-modifying antirheumatic drugs: 2013 update. Ann Rheum Dis. 2014;73(3):492–509.
54. Singh JA, Saag KG, Bridges L Jr, Akl EA, Bannuru RR, Sullivan MC et al (2015) American College of Rheumatology guidelines for the treatment of rheumatoid arthritis. Arthritis Care Res 2015:1–15
55. Smolen JS, van der Heijde D, Machold KP, Aletaha D, Landewe R (2014) Proposal for a new nomenclature of disease modifying anti-rheumatic drugs. Ann Rheum Dis 73:3–5
56. Gaujoux-Viala C, Smolen JS, Landewe R, Dougados M, Kvien TK, Mola EM et al (2010) Current evidence for the management of rheumatoid arthritis with synthetic disease modifying antirheumatic drugs:a systematic literature review informing the EULAR recommendations for the management of rheumatoid arthritis. Ann Rheum Dis 69(6):1004–1009
57. Gaujoux-Viala C, Nam J, Ramiro S, Landewe R, Buch MH, Smolen JS et al (2014) Efficacy of conventional synthetic disease modifying antirheumatic drugs, glucocorticoids and tofacitinib: a systematic review informing the 2013 update of the EULAR recommendations for management of rheumatoid arthritis. Ann Rheum Dis 73(3):510–515
58. Chan ESL, Fernandez P, Cronstein BN (2007) Methotrexate in rheumatoid arthritis. Expert Rev Clin Immunol 3(1):27–33
59. Rachapalli SM, Williams R, Walsh DA, Young A, Kiely PDW, Choy E et al (2010) First-line DMARD choice in early rheumatoid arthritis – do prognostic factors play a role? Rheumatology 49(7):1267–1271
60. Kumar P, Banik S (2013) Pharmacotherapy options in rheumatoid arthritis. Clin Med Insights Arthritis Musculoskelet Disord 6:35–43
61. Chan ESL, Cronstein BN (2013) Mechanism of action of methotrexate. Bull Hosp Jt Dis 71(Suppl 1):S5–S8
62. American College of Rheumatology Adhoc Committee on Clinical Guidelines (1996) Guidelines for management of rheumatoid arthritis. Arthritis Rheum 39:713–722
63. American College of Rheumatology Subcommittee on Rheumatoid Arthritis Guidelines (2002) Guidelines for the management of rheumatoid arthritis: 2002 update. Arthritis Rheum 46:328–346
64. Jones KW, Patel SR (2000) A Family Physician's guide to monitoring methotrexate. Am Fam Physician 62:1607–1612

65. Hoekstram M, Haagsma C, Neef C, Proost J, Knuif A, van de Laar M (2004) Bioavailability of higher dose methotrexate comparing oral dose methotrexate and subcutaneous administration in patients with rheumatoid arthritis. J Rheumatol 31(4):645–648

66. Yazici Y, Bata Y (2013) Parenteral methotrexate for treatment of rheumatoid arthritis. Bull Hosp Jt Dis 71(Suppl 1):46–48

67. Cipriani P, Ruscitti P, Carubbi F, Liakouli V, Giacomelli R (2014) Methotrexate in rheumatoid arthritis: optimising therapy among different formulations. Current and emerging paradigms. Clin Ther 36(3):427–435

68. Schiff MH, Jaffe JS, Freundlich B (2014) Head-to-head, randomised, crossover study of oral versus subcutaneous methotrexate in patients with rheumatoid arthritis: drug exposure limitations of oral methotrexate at doses >15mg may be overcome with subcutaneous administration. Ann Rheum Dis 73(8):1549–1551

69. Sharma P, Scott DGI (2015) Optimising methotrexate therapy in rheumatoid arthritis: the case of subcutaneous methotrexate prior to biologics. Drugs 75(17):1953–1956

70. van Ede AE, Laan RFJM, Rood MJ, Huizinga TWJ, van de Laar MAFJ, van Denderen CJ et al (2001) Effect of folic or folinic acid supplementation on the toxicity and efficacy of methotrexate in rheumatoid arthritis. Arthritis Rheum 44:1515–1524

71. Whittle SL, Hughes RA (2004) Folate supplementation and methotrexate treatment in rheumatoid arthritis: a review. Rheumatology 43(3):267–271

72. Shea B, Swinden MV, Ghogomu ET, Ortiz Z, Katchamart W, Rader T et al (2014) Folic acid and folinic acid for reducing side effects in patients receiving methotrexate for rheumatoid arthritis. J Rheumatol 41(6):1049–1060

73. Eaton AT, Davis PN, Ndefo UA, Ebiogwu A (2013) Update on pharmacotherapeutic options for rheumatoid arthritis. US Pharmacist 38(10):44–48

74. Breedveld FC, Dayer JM (2000) Leflunomide: mode of action in the treatment of rheumatoid arthritis. Ann Rheum Dis 59(11):841–849

75. Rozman B (2002) Clinical pharmacokinetics of leflunomide. Clin Pharmacokinet 41:421–430

76. Maddison P, Kiely P, Kirkham B, Lawson T, Moots R, Proudfoot D et al (2005) Leflunomide in rheumatoid arthritis: recommendations through a process of consensus. Rheumatology 44:280–286

77. Ben-Zvi I, Kivity S, Langevitz P, Shoenfeld Y (2012) Hydroxychloroquine: from malaria to autoimmunity. Clin Rev Allergy Immunol 42(2):145–153

78. Silva JC, Mariz HA, Rocha LF Jr, Oliveira PS, Dantas AT, Duarte AL et al (2013) Hydroxychloroquine decreases Th17-related cytokines in systemic lupus erythematosus and rheumatoid arthritis patients. Clinics 68(6):766–771

79. Al-Bari MA (2015) Chloroquine analogues in drug discovery: new directions of uses, mechanisms of actions and toxic manifestations from malaria to multifarious disease. Antimicrob Chemother 70(6):1608–1621

80. Landewe RB, Goei The HS, van Rijthoven AW, Breedveld FC, Dijkmans BA (1994) A randomised double blind 24 week controlled study of low dose ciclosporin versus chloroquine for early rheumatoid arthritis. Arthritis Rheum 37:637–643

81. Ledingham J, Deighton C (2005) Update on the British Society for Rheumatology guidelines for prescribing TNF-alfa blockers in adults with rheumatoid arthritis (update of previous guidelines of April 2001). Rheumatology 44:157–163

82. Ding T, Ledingham J, Luqmani R, Westlake S, Hyrich K, Lunt M et al (2010) BSR and BHPR rheumatoid arthritis guidelines on safety of anti-TNF therapies. Rheumatology 49:2217–2219

83. Curis JR, Singh JA (2011) The use of biologics in rheumatoid arthritis: current and emerging paradigms of care. Clin Ther 33(6):679–707

84. Singh JA, Cameron C, Noorbaloochi S, Cullis T, Tucker M, Christensen R et al (2015) Risk of serious infection in biological treatment of patients with rheumatoid arthritis: a systematic review and meta-analysis. Lancet 386:258–265

85. Ruderman EM (2012) Overview of safety of non-biologic and biologic DMARDs. Rheumatology 51(Suppl 6):vi37–vi43

86. Malaviya AP, Ledingham J, Bloxham J, Bosworth A, Buch M, Choy E et al (2014) The 2013 BSR and BHPR guideline for the use of intravenous tocilizumab in the treatment of adult patients with rheumatoid arthritis. Rheumatology 53(7):1344–1346

87. Mariette X, Matucci-Cerinic M, Pavelka K, Taylor P, van Vollenhoven R, Heatley R et al (2011) Malignancies associated with tumour necrosis factor inhibitors in registries and prospective observational studies: a systematic review and meta-analysis. Ann Rheum Dis 70(11):1895–1904

88. Le Blay P, Mouterde G, Barnetche T, Morel J, Combe B (2012) Risk of malignancy including non-melanoma skin cancers with anti-tumour necrosis factor therapy in patients with rheumatoid arthritis: meta-analysis of registries and systematic review of long term extension studies. Clin Exp Rheumatol 30(5):756–764

89. Cush JJ, Kay J, Dao KH (2012) Does rheumatoid arthritis or biologic therapy increase cancer risk? Drug Safety Quart 4(2):1–2

90. Lopez-Olivo MA, Tavar JH, Martinez-Lopez JA, Pollono EN, Cueto JP, Gonzales-Crespo MR et al (2012) Risk of malignancies in patients with rheumatoid arthritis treated with biologic therapy: a meta-analysis. JAMA 308(9):898–908

91. Lis K, Kuzawinka O, Balkowiec-Iskra E (2014) Tumour necrosis factor inhibitors – state of knowledge. Arch Med Sci 10(6):1175–1185

92. Codreanu C, Damjanov N (2015) Safety of biologics in rheumatoid arthritis: data from randomized controlled trials and registries. Biologics 9:1–6

93. Bukhari M, Abernethy R, Deighton C, Ding T, Hyrich K, Lunt M et al (2011) BSR and BHPR guidelines on the use of rituximab in rheumatoid arthritis. Rheumatology 50(12):2311–2313

94. Emery P, Breedveld FC, Lemmel EM, Katwasser JP, Dawes PT, Gomor B et al (2000) A comparison of the efficacy and safety of leflunomide and methotrexate for the treatment of rheumatoid arthritis. Rheumatology 39(6):655–665

95. Singer O, Gibofsky A (2011) Methotrexate versus leflunomide in rheumatoid arthritis: what is new in 2011? Curr Opin Rheumatol 23(3):288–292

96. Hider SL, Silman A, Bunn D, Manning S, Symmons D, Lunt M (2006) Comparing the long term clinical outcome of treatment with methotrexate or sulfasalazine prescribed as the first disease-modifying antirheumatic drug in patients with inflammatory polyarthritis. Ann Rheum Dis 65(11):1449–1455

97. Lie E, Uhlig T, van der Heijde D, Rodevand E, Kalstad S, Kaufmann C et al (2012) Effectiveness of sulfasalazine and methotrexate in 1102 DMARD-naive patients with early RA. Rheumatology 51(4):670–678

98. Cheung JM, Scarsbrook D, Klinkhoff AV (2012) Characterisation of patients with arthritis referred for gold therapy in the era of biologics. J Rheumatol 39(4):716–719

99. Lee ATY, Pile K (2003) Disease modifying antirheumatic drugs in adult rheumatoid arthritis. Aust Prescr 26:36–40

100. Temprano KK, Bandlamudi R, Moore TL (2005) Antirheumatic drugs in pregnancy and lactation. Semin Arthritis Rheum 35(2):112–121

101. Ostensen M, Forger F (2009) Management of RA medications in pregnant patients. Nat Rev Rheumatol 5(7):382–290

102. Makol A, Wright K, Amin S (2011) Rheumatoid arthritis and pregnancy: safety considerations in pharmacological management. Drugs 71(5):1973–1987

103. Partlett R, Roussou E (2011) The treatment of rheumatoid arthritis during pregnancy. Rheumatol Int 31(4):445–449

104. Ostensen M, Forger F (2013) How safe are anti-rheumatic drugs during pregnancy? Curr Opin Pharmacol 13(3):470–475

105. Sammaritano LR, Bermas BL (2014) Rheumatoid arthritis medications and lactation. Curr Opin Rheumatol 26(3):354–360

106. Flint J, Panchal S, Hurrell A, van de Venne M, Gayed M, Schreiber K et al (2016) BSR and BHPR guideline on prescribing drugs in pregnancy and breastfeeding-Part I: standard and biologic disease modifying anti-rheumatic drugs and corticosteroids. Rheumatology. doi:10.1093/rheumatology/kev404

107. Skorpen G, Hoeltzenbeing M, Tincani A, Fischer-Betz R, Elefant E, Chambers C et al (2016) The EULAR points to consider for use of antirheumatic drugs before pregnancy, and during pregnancy and lactation. Ann Rheum Dis 75:795–810. doi:10.1136/annrheumdis-2015-208840

108. Azzopardi L (2007) Developing a pharmaceutical care plan for patients with rheumatoid arthritis. MPhil Dissertation Department of Pharmaceutical Sciences. University of Strathclyde, Glasgow

Chapter 3
Pharmacoeconomics and Rheumatoid Arthritis

Maurice Zarb Adami and Bernard Coleiro

3.1 Introduction

Pharmacoeconomics refers to the scientific discipline that compares the value of one pharmaceutical drug or drug therapy to another. It is a subdiscipline of health economics. How do health, pharmacy, medications and financial constraints impact on each other? What are the consequences of innovative drug development and expensive medications? Does quality of life and health come at a cost? This chapter attempts to delve into the aspects of pharmacoeconomics and presents case scenarios of pharmacoeconomic analysis within rheumatoid arthritis.

3.2 Health as a Human Right

Every human being, by virtue of being so, enjoys a number of human rights that are inalienable (cannot be given away), universal (apply everywhere) and egalitarian (apply equally to all). These rights are listed in the Universal Declaration of Human Rights (UDHR), which is ratified by 192 countries and includes the right to life, liberty and security of person [1]. Specifically, Article 25 of the UDHR states that "Everyone has the right to a standard of living adequate for the health and well-being of himself and of his family, including food, clothing, housing and

M. Zarb Adami, PhD (✉)
Department of Pharmacy, Faculty of Medicine and Surgery, University of Malta, Msida, Malta
e-mail: maurice.zarb-adami@um.edu.mt

B. Coleiro, MD, FRCP, MPhil (Melit) (✉)
Faculty of Medicine and Surgery, University of Malta, Msida, Malta

Department of Medicine, Mater Dei Hospital, Msida, Malta
e-mail: bernardcoleiro454@gmail.com

© Springer Science+Business Media Singapore 2016
L. Grech, A. Lau (eds.), *Pharmaceutical Care Issues of Patients with Rheumatoid Arthritis*, DOI 10.1007/978-981-10-1421-5_3

medical care and necessary social services, and the right to security in the event of unemployment, sickness, disability, widowhood, old age or other lack of livelihood in circumstances beyond his control".

3.2.1 Health at a Price?

All will agree that the best things in life are free. It is a pity, however, that the next best things are expensive. In the vast majority of cases man is born healthy, but as time goes by, man is susceptible to a wide spectrum of diseases ranging from a slight inconvenience such as common cold to more serious and often fatal conditions such as cancer. Man is born with a number of basic instincts which enable him to face the environment and develop into maturity. Food, reproduction, health, money and society are the main drivers which man, mostly unconsciously, uses. These are mirrored by the industries that have developed over time. The health industry is a combination of goods and services that treat patients who need diagnostic, surgical, therapeutic, preventive, rehabilitative and palliative care. These are delivered in a variety of ways. Basic community services are provided by family doctors and community pharmacists, whilst specialised services are provided in ad hoc centres, namely, hospitals. These goods and services are not free. They may be delivered without charge at the point of delivery, but all are paid for, whether by the individual, the government or insurance companies.

3.2.2 Health Services and Economic Implications

The provision of health services is an economic activity. Health is frequently not appreciated by an individual and is taken for granted. However, if the state of health is lost, then it becomes pressing on the individual to find means to regain his healthy state if he is to self-preserve. Apart from the individual, society itself is a stakeholder in the health of its members. Sick people do not contribute to the economies of their society but instead are a drain on such economies. Governments realise that health systems are very important to the people themselves. In democracies, members of government must attract the people's approval, through votes, on a recurrent basis. Parties running for elections are always keen to attract votes, and promising improvements in the delivery of health services proves to be a very good vote catcher. There are a number of factors driving the demand for increased expenditure on healthcare. Advances in all aspects of medical science and technology (such as through development and use of innovative antibiotics, anaesthesia, diagnostics and monoclonal antibodies) have saved the lives of a number of patients who would otherwise have died prematurely. These advances are very expensive. However, these advances enable us to treat conditions that were previously untreatable.

Research and medicine have led the way to people living longer, but longevity has its own economic implications [2–9]. The problem of successfully treating and saving more people also means having more of the population in advanced age and this is the problem of success. Having the population live to a ripe old age has a consequence that they are subject to diseases of old age or to diseases they would not have acquired had they died of other conditions at an earlier age. This is called the problem of success. The baby boom following the Second World War combined with a reduction in early mortality results in a large percentage of the population going over retirement age, leading to increasing demands on pensions as well healthcare costs [10–13].

As time goes by, expectations continue to increase, fuelled by increasing elderly populations, increased information via the internet, improved technologies and the ability to treat conditions that until recently were considered untreatable. In order to provide the health facilities that are required by society, resources must be made available. Unfortunately, resources are finite, and there are many other societal activities vying for a share of the available resources, including education, policing, pensions and housing. Competition for ever decreasing resources means that the evaluation of healthcare goods and services must go beyond considerations of safety and efficacy and that healthcare practitioners must take into account the economic impact of these goods and services on the cost of healthcare. A challenge for healthcare professionals is to continue to provide quality patient care whilst making best use of the minimal resources available.

3.2.3 Pharmacoeconomic Implications

Pharmacoeconomics basically involves the process of identifying, measuring and comparing the costs, risks and benefits of programmes, services or therapies so as to establish which alternative produces the best health outcome for the resource invested. This means weighing the cost of providing particular pharmacy products against the consequences (outcomes) achieved by using those products, to ascertain which of the alternatives yields the optimal outcome per dollar spent, in other words, most bang for the buck. This information guides clinicians in choosing the most cost-effective treatment options. The research may be carried out from different points of view, and this can give different results. Common perspectives include those of the patient, provider, payer and society.

3.3 The Mutlifacets of Cost

In areas as complicated as medical treatment, many different types of cost come into play and they must all be taken into consideration. The costs of any therapy or procedure may be or include:

- Direct medical costs such as medications, supplies such as dressings and syringes, laboratory tests, scans, bed-space and professional time.
- Direct non-medical costs such as food, transport, family care and home aides.
- Indirect non-medical costs, i.e. the costs of reduced productivity. These costs result from morbidity and mortality and are an important source of resource consumption, especially from the perspective of the patient. Morbidity implies lost wages due to absence from work and mortality refers to income foregone due to early death.
- Intangible costs such as pain, suffering, inconvenience and grief.
- Opportunity costs, i.e. revenue foregone from inability to perform other procedures with the financial resources utilised in this case.
- Incremental costs, that is, the cost to produce one more unit of outcome benefit.

The outcomes or consequences of a condition and its treatment are an important consideration of pharmacoeconomic analyses, and like costs, they may be classified. The ECHO model places outcomes into one of three categories: economic, clinical and humanistic [14]. Economic outcomes are the direct, indirect and intangible costs compared with the consequences of medical treatment alternatives. Clinical outcomes are the medical events that occur as a result of disease or treatment (such as safety and efficacy endpoints). Humanistic outcomes are the consequences of disease or treatment on patient functional status or quality of life along several dimensions (such as physical function, social function, general health and well-being, and life satisfaction).

Outcomes may also be classified as positive or negative. Positive outcomes include a desired effect of a drug (efficacy or effectiveness measure), measured as cases cured, life-years gained or improved health-related quality of life (HRQOL). A negative outcome is an undesired or adverse effect of a drug, possibly manifested as a treatment failure, an adverse drug reaction (ADR), a drug toxicity or even death. Outcomes can also be as intermediate or final. Intermediate outcomes can serve as a proxy for more appropriate final outcomes. Obtaining a reduction in low-density lipoprotein (LDL) cholesterol levels with a lipid-lowering agent is an intermediate consequence that is used as a proxy for a more meaningful final outcome such as a lower cardiovascular problems including lower myocardial infarction rate in rheumatoid arthritis patient population Intermediate consequences are frequently used in pharmacoeconomic analyses because they are more readily measured and their use reduces the cost and time required to conduct a trial. Pharmacoeconomic evaluations may be partial or full. Partial economic evaluations may be simple presentations of outcomes or resources consumed and thus require a minimum of time and effort. If only the consequences or only the costs of a programme, service or treatment are described, the evaluation becomes an outcome or cost description.

3.3.1 Cost-Consequence Analysis

A cost-outcome or cost-consequence analysis (CCA) describes the costs and consequences of an alternative but does not provide a comparison with other treatment options. Another example of a partial evaluation is a cost analysis that compares the costs of two or more alternatives but without regard to outcome. On the other hand, full economic evaluations include cost-minimisation, cost-benefit, cost-effectiveness and cost-utility analyses. Each method is used to compare at least two competing programmes or treatment alternatives. The methods are all similar in the way they measure cost (in dollars) but differ in their measurement of outcomes.

3.3.2 Cost-Minimisation Analysis

Cost-minimisation analysis (CMA) involves the determination of the least costly alternative when comparing two or more treatment alternatives which are equivalent in safety and efficacy (i.e. the two alternatives must be equivalent therapeutically). Once this equivalency is established, the costs can be identified, measured and compared in monetary units (dollars). If therapeutic equivalence has not been proven, then this comparison would not be valid. CMA is a relatively straightforward and simple method for comparing competing programmes or treatment alternatives with identical therapeutic profiles. If two drugs are used for the same condition, say methotrexate and leflunomide, and have been documented as equivalent in effectiveness and rate of side effects, then the costs of using these drugs could be compared using CMA. These costs should extend beyond a mere comparison of drug acquisition costs but should include the preparation (pharmacist and technician time), administration (nursing time) and storage. If appropriate, other costs to be valued may include the cost of physician visits, number of hospital days and pharmacokinetic consultations, for example, blood level monitoring. The least expensive agent, considering all these costs, should be chosen. This method is used frequently, especially when comparing originator with relevant generic products. In CMA, costs are measured in monetary units (USD, Euros, Yen), and outcomes are measured in clinical units.

3.3.3 Cost-Effectiveness Analysis

Cost-effectiveness analysis (CEA) is used to summarise the health benefits resulting from the resources used by competing therapies so as to enable clinicians and policymakers to choose among them. CEA involves comparing programmes or treatment alternatives with different safety and efficacy profiles. The results of CEA are usually expressed as a ratio—either as an average cost-effectiveness ratio (ACER) or as an incremental cost-effectiveness ratio (ICER). An ACER represents the total cost of a programme or treatment alternative divided by its clinical outcome to yield a ratio representing the dollar cost per specific clinical outcome gained, independent of comparators. The ACER can be summarised as follows:

$$ACER = \frac{\textbf{Healthcare costs}\,(\text{in }\$)}{\textbf{Clinical outcome}\,(\text{in clinical units})}$$

This allows the costs and outcomes to be reduced to a single value to allow for comparison. Using this ratio, the clinician would choose the alternative with the least cost per outcome gained. As explained above, one ACER does not make a full economic exercise, and two ACERs must be compared for this to be achieved.

Generally speaking, increased clinical effectiveness is gained at an increased cost. Is the increased benefit always worth the increased cost? For example, if antibiotic A will clear an infection in 7 days at a cost of 20 USD, is it worth using antibiotic B which clears the infection in 5 days but costs 25 USD?

Incremental CEA may be used to determine the additional cost and effectiveness gained when one treatment alternative is compared with the next best treatment alternative. In this case, instead of comparing the ACERs of each treatment alternative, the additional cost that a treatment alternative imposes over another treatment is compared with the additional effect, benefit or outcome it provides. This is called the ICER.

$$ICER = \frac{\textbf{Cost}_A\,(\$) - \textbf{Cost}_B\,(\$)}{\textbf{Benefit}_A - \textbf{Benefit}_B}$$

In CEA, cost is measured in dollars, and outcomes are measured in terms of obtaining a specific therapeutic outcome. These outcomes are often expressed in physical units, natural units or nonmonetary units (lives saved, cases cured, life expectancy or drop in blood pressure).

3.3.4   Cost-Benefit Analysis

Cost-benefit analysis (CBA) is used for the identification, measurement and comparison of the benefits and costs of one or more programmes (or treatment alternatives). What will be the expenditure on a breast screening programme and what would be the expenditure on a colorectal screening programme? What health benefits for the community would result from either of these two programmes? CBAs are also performed on non-medical projects, e.g. would a bridge or a tunnel provide the best option at a particular location? Costs and benefits can be expressed as a ratio (a benefit-to-cost ratio), a net benefit or a net cost. A wise administrator would choose the programme which gives the highest net benefit or the greatest benefit-to-cost (B/C) ratio.

A B/C ratio greater than 1 indicates that the programme should be carried out, as the benefits to be realised outweigh the cost of providing it. If the B/C ratio is equal to 1, the benefits equal the cost and no advantage is gained by undertaking it. If the B/C ratio is less than 1, then the cost of providing the programme or treatment alternative outweighs the benefits realised by it.

CBAs should be employed when evaluating alternatives in which the costs and benefits do not occur simultaneously. CBAs may be used when comparing programmes with different objectives because all benefits are converted into dollars. Another aspect to be kept in mind when carrying out CBAs is the magnitude of the benefit/benefits obtained. A B/C ratio of 100 would seem attractive enough on its own, but a 100 % increase of 1000 USD is still only 1000 USD, whilst a 100 % increase on a spend of 1million USD would give a hundred million in return.

In cost-benefit assessments, both costs and benefits are measured in monetary units. However, valuing health benefits in monetary terms can be difficult and controversial.

3.3.5   Cost-Utility Analysis

Cost-utility analysis (CUA) is used for comparing treatment alternatives that incorporate patient preferences and HRQOL in the method used. CUA can compare cost, quality and the quantity of patient-years. Cost is measured in dollars, and therapeutic outcome is measured in patient-weighted utilities rather than in physical units. Often the utility measurement used is a quality-adjusted life-year (QALY) gained. QALY is a common measure of health status used in CUA, combining morbidity and mortality data.

Life-years gained (LYG) is a respected outcome from a clinical perspective, but quality-adjusted life-years (QALYs) gained are very important to the patients themselves. A number of measures of health-related quality of live (HRQOLs) have been developed such as the SF-36 and the DAS-28.

3.3.6   The Cost of Relative Risk, Absolute Risk and Numbers Needed to Treat

Clinical trials frequently present results as the reduction in risk of an adverse event occurring by the administration of an active ingredient to a treated group of patients as against the risk of the same event occurring in a control group who receive a placebo. The result can appear to be impressive, especially as it is usually the relative risk reduction which is reported, rather than the absolute risk. Suppose that a group of 5000 patients with hyperlipidaemia were enrolled in a study, with 2500 being a drug under test and the other 2500 being given a placebo over a 2-year period. Suppose further that of the treated group 56 patients suffered an untoward event (myocardial infarction, fatal or non-fatal or death), whilst in the placebo group 84 patients had a similar outcome. The event rate is calculated as a ratio of events in the group over number of patients in the group.

$$Event\,rate = \frac{Events\,in\,group}{No\,of\,patients\,in\,group}$$

$$Event\,rate\,(ctrl) = \frac{84}{2500} = 0.0336 * 100 = 3.36\%$$

$$Event\,rate\,(trtd) = \frac{56}{2500} = 0.0224 * 100 = 2.24\%$$

Ctrl, control group; trtd, treated group

The relative risk reduction is defined as the treated event reduction as a percentage of the event rate in the control group.

$$Relative\,risk\,reduction = \frac{Event\,rate\,(trtd) - Event\,rate\,(ctrl)}{Event\,rate\,(ctrl)} * 100$$

$$Relative\,risk\,reduction = \frac{0.0336 - 0.0224}{0.0336} * 100 = 33.33\%$$

The absolute risk reduction is defined as the difference in the event rates between the control group and the treated group.

$$Absolute\,risk\,reduction = 0.0336 - 0.0224 = 0.0112 * 100 = 1.12\%$$

On the other hand, the number needed to treat (NNTT) is defined as the number of patients who must be treated in order to prevent the occurrence of one event, or for one patient to achieve the benefit. This is the inverse of the absolute risk reduction.

$$Number\,needed\,to\,treat = 1 / 0.0112 = 89.28$$

Therefore, one needs to treat 90 patients to achieve one untoward event less than would be expected from untreated patients. The cost of that one less untoward event is the cost of treating 90 patients for a 2-year period. The same concept can be applied to determine the number needed to harm (NNTH), that is the number of patients that need to be treated before one adverse effect surfaces.

3.4 Applying Pharmacoeconomics to Rheumatoid Arthritis

Pharmacoeconomics is a useful tool to therapeutic committees in their role of drawing up formularies and protocols to ensure that the use of sometimes very expensive drugs is carried out in an economic, effective and equitable manner. A sample of three different pharmacoeconomic studies carried out in research has been selected for some consideration in this chapter to outline a few examples.

3.4.1   Case Study 1

As outlined in Chap. 1, rheumatoid arthritis patients frequently suffer from co-morbidities. Rheumatoid arthritis patients suffering from coronary artery disease are administered statin. A study carried out by Bansback et al. examined the impact of the therapies on cardiovascular disease and rheumatoid arthritis over time [15]. The base-case scenario considered female patients whilst a 10-year horizon was adopted. The authors stated that the perspective was that of the US healthcare payer. The key clinical parameters were the number of CHD events and the response to statin therapy, which was measured by the rheumatoid arthritis Disease Activity Score (DAS28). The measure of benefit was the number of quality-adjusted life-years (QALYs) gained and these were discounted at an annual rate of 5%. The analysis considered the direct medical costs of the acquisition of the statins and the treatment of rheumatoid arthritis (other drugs, out-patient visits, health professionals, diagnostic tests and hospitalisation).

Over 10 years, the incremental cost of statin therapy ($62,046) over no statin therapy ($57,356) was $4,690. The mean gain in QALYs with statin therapy (3.38) over no statin therapy (2.94) was 0.44. The incremental cost-effectiveness ratio of statin therapy, over no therapy, was $10,650 per QALY gained.

The authors concluded that statin therapy could be highly cost-effective for the treatment of rheumatoid arthritis patients due to its dual effects in reducing the risk of coronary artery disease.

3.4.2   Case Study 2

This study consists of a review of 29 randomised controlled trials and is included because it illustrates the use of number needed to treat (NNTT), as well as the use of the incremental cost-effectiveness ratio (ICER) in the determination of cost-effectiveness. This report reviews the clinical effectiveness and cost-effectiveness of adalimumab, etanercept and infliximab, agents that inhibit tumour necrosis factor-α (TNF-α), when used in the treatment of rheumatoid arthritis (RA) in adults [16].

Table 3.1 Summary of results obtained by Chen et al. indicating NNTTs to achieve various ACRs

	Adalimumab	Etanercept	Infliximab
ACR 20	3.6 (3.1–4.2)	2.1 (1.9–2.4)	3.2 (2.7–4.0)
ACR 50	4.2 (3.7–5.0)	3.1 (2.7–3.6)	5.0 (3.8–6.7)
ACR 70	7.7 (5.9–11.1)	7.7 (6.3–10.0)	11.1 (7.7–20.0)

The numbers needed to treat (NNTs) (95 % CI) required to produce an American College for Rheumatology (ACR) response compared with placebo are reproduced in Table 3.1.

The authors report that the ICER for etanercept used last is £24,000 per QALY, substantially lower than for adalimumab (£30,000 per QALY) or for infliximab (£38,000 per QALY). First-line use as monotherapy generates ICERs around £50,000 per QALY for adalimumab and etanercept. Using the combination of methotrexate and a TNF-α inhibitor as first-line treatment generates much higher ICERs, as it precludes subsequent use of methotrexate alone, which is cheap. The ICERs for sequential use are of the same order as using the TNF-α inhibitor alone.

3.4.3   Case Study 3

This was a 6-month study undertaken to determine the improved QOL and the incremental cost-effectiveness ratio (ICER) involved in treating Maltese patients suffering from resistant RA, with TNF-α inhibitors [17]. The high costs of the new DMARDs elicited the need to carry out pharmacoeconomical assessments in order to inform policy- and decisionmakers of their cost-effectiveness. The 13 patients included had failed to achieve a low disease activity despite traditional DMARD/s therapy and were switched onto a TNF-α inhibitor (etanercept, adalimumab or infliximab). Patients were not eligible to participate if pregnant or planning to conceive suffering from TB or hep B and if they are diagnosed with juvenile chronic arthritis, ankylosing spondylitis, osteoarthritis, psoriatic arthritis and/or any other rheumatological condition.

The disease-specific Health Assessment Questionnaire (HAQ), the generic SF-36 and the DAS28 were used as outcome measures. This prospective study, carried out between 2010 and 2011, had a time phase of 6 months, during which patients were assessed 3 times through the SF-36 and HAQ. At phase 1 (t-0 months), patients were still being treated with conventional DMARD therapy. Subjects who accepted to participate in the study were interviewed by the investigator using the HAQ and SF-36. Raw data obtained for both the SF-36 and the HAQ were inputted in a Microsoft Excel Database. The final HAQ score and summary scores for every

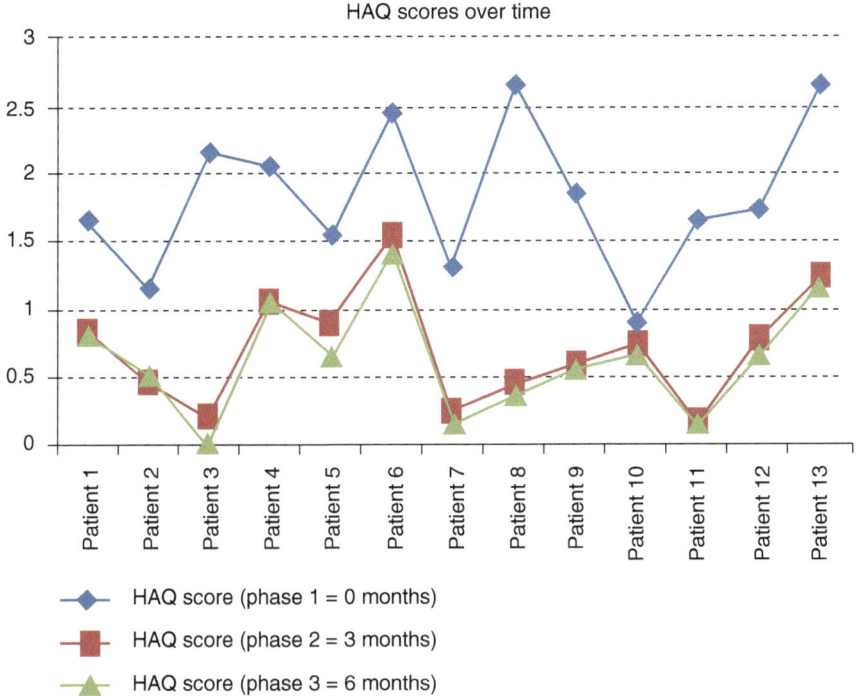

Fig. 3.1 Illustration of the HAQ scores reported by patients at baseline, 3 months and 6 months following TNF-α inhibitor therapy

SF-36 domain were calculated. At phase 2 (t-3 months after initiation of TNF-α inhibitor therapy), participants were reinterviewed using the same questionnaires. At phase 3 (t-6 months), data from the SF-36 and HAQ were again collected following 6 months of TNF-α inhibitor therapy. During both phases 1 and 3, patients were examined by the rheumatology consultant and assigned a DAS-28 score as a measure of disease activity. In both phases, medical case notes of patients were reviewed and related data were collected, namely, DAS-28 scores, treatment regimens, adverse events, history of hospitalisation during the study period and surgeries performed related to RA (Figs. 3.1, 3.2 and 3.3).

The three figures illustrate the improvement achieved in each of the measures utilised in this study from the utilisation of the TNF-α inhibitor therapy.

The study concludes that an improvement in quality of life is achieved within 6 months of therapy, and if this is sustained, the magnitude of the pharmacoeconomic impact increases substantially. This data transmits the message that, for each individual patient, the potential of improving the quality of life and the pharmacoeconomic benefit is evident. Long-term benefit of biological treatment can be evaluated through further assessments.

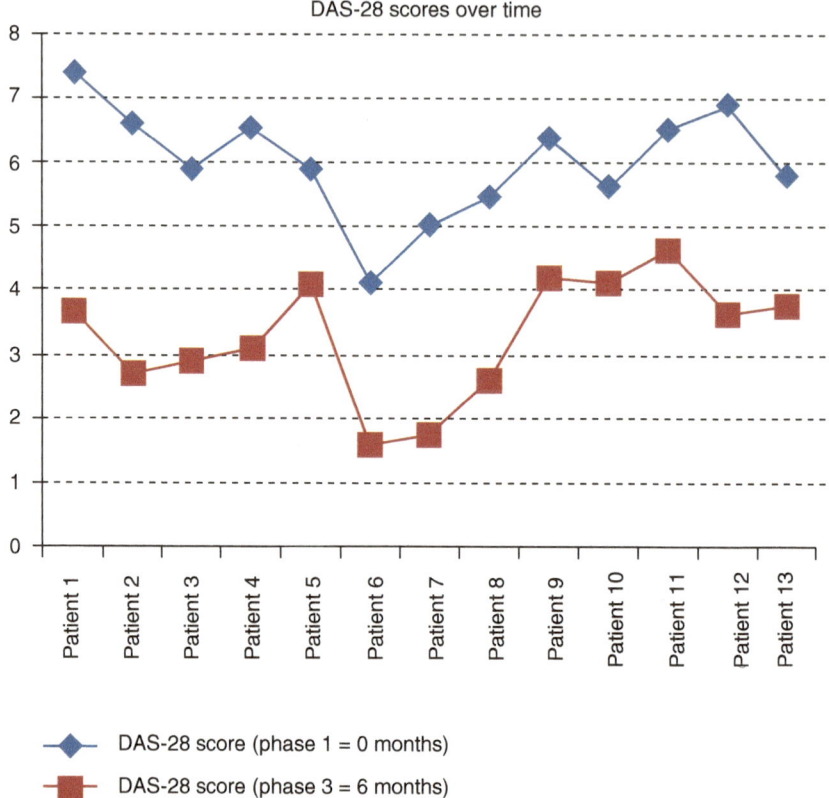

Fig. 3.2 Illustration of the DAS-28 scores reported by every patient at baseline (prior to initiation of TNF-α inhibitor therapy) and at phase 3 (6 months after initiation of TNF-α inhibitor therapy)

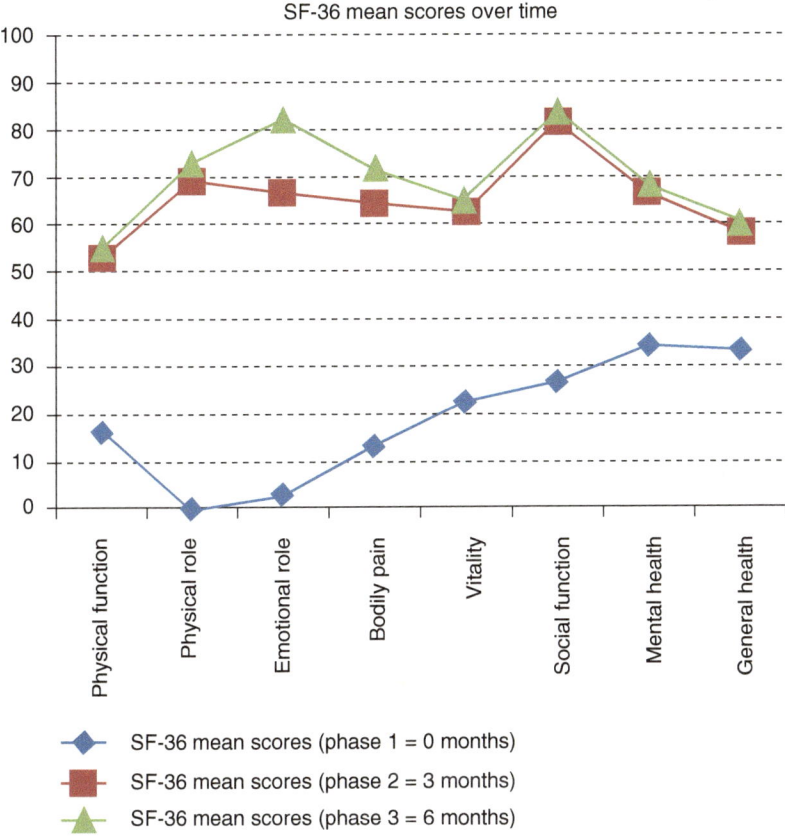

Fig. 3.3 Illustration of the scores for every domain within the SF-36 at baseline, 3 months and 6 months following TNF-α inhibitor therapy

Take Home Messages
- All health services are paid for, whether these are paid for directly by the individual patients, the society through tax, the governments or insurance companies.
- The advent of medical technology has resulted in more conditions being treated leading to increased life expectancy and longevity.
- The baby boom is at the moment adding to an increased ageing population.
- Community pharmacists are often the first port of call to patients in the community setting.
- The longevity and ageing population result in economic constraints on the healthcare costs.
- Pharmacoeconomics is the subspecialty of health economics which takes into account the different types of costs, outcomes and impact on the quality of life of patients helping clinicians and policymakers to choose the most cost-effective pharmacotherapy whilst maintaining an optimum individualised quality of care.

References

1. United Nations General Assembly (1948) Universal declaration of human rights. 217A(III). http://www.refworld.org/docid/3ae6b3712c.html. Accessed 21 Feb 2016
2. Spillman BC, Lubitz J (2000) The effect of longevity on spending for acute and long-term care. N Engl J Med 342(19):1409–1415
3. Rice DP, Fineman N (2004) Economic implications of increased longevity in the United States. Annu Rev Public Health 25:457–473
4. Vladeck BC (2005) Economic and policy implications of improving longevity. J Am Geriatr Soc 53(9s):S304–S307
5. Strunk BC, Ginsburg PB, Banker MI (2006) The effect of population ageing on future hospital demand. Health Aff 25(3):w141–w149
6. Goldman DP, Cutler D, Rowe JW, Michaud PC, Sullivan J, Peneva D et al (2013) Substantial health and economic returns from delayed aging may warrant a new focus for medical research. Health Aff 32(10):1698–1705
7. Bloom DE, Chatterji S, Kowal P, Lloyd-Sherlock P, McKee M, Rechel B et al (2015) Macroeconomic implication of population ageing and selected policy responses. Lancet 385(9968):649–657
8. Prince M, Wu F, Guo Y, Gutierrez Robledo LM, O'Donnell M, Sullivan R et al (2015) The burden of disease in older people and implications for health policy and practice. Lancet 385(9967):549–562
9. Suzman R, Beard JR, Boerman T, Chatterji S (2015) Health in an ageing world – what do we know? Lancet 385(9967):484–486
10. Reinhardt UE (2000) Healthcare for the ageing baby boom: lessons learnt from abroad. J Econ Perspect 14(2):71–83
11. Knickman JR, Snell EK (2002) The 2030 problem: caring for ageing baby boomers. Health Serv Res 37(4):849–884
12. Garrett N, Martini M (2007) The boomers are coming: a total cost of care model of the impact population ageing on the cost of chronic conditions in the United States. Dis Manag 10(2):51–60
13. Keehan S, Sisko A, Truffer C, Smith S, Cowan C, Poissal J et al (2008) Health spending projections through 2017: the baby-boom generation is coming to Medicare. Health Aff 27(2):w145–w155
14. Kozma CM, Reeder CE, Shulz RM (1993) Economic, clinical and humanistic outcomes: a planning model for pharmacoeconomic research. Clin Ther 15(6):1121–1132
15. Bansback N, Ara R, Ward S, Anis A, Choi HK (2009) Statin therapy in rheumatoid arthritis: a cost-effectiveness and value of information analysis. Pharmacoeconomics 27(1):25–37
16. Chen YF, Jobanputra P, Barton P, Jowett S, Bryan S, Clark W et al (2006) A systematic review of the effectiveness of adalimumab, etanercept and infliximab for the treatment of rheumatoid arthritis in adults and an economic evaluation of their cost-effectiveness. Health Technol Assess 10(42):iii–iv, xi–xiii, 1–229
17. Coleiro B (2009) Cost effectiveness of drugs which suppress the rheumatic disease process. M. Phil dissertation. Department of Pharmacy. University of Malta, Msida

Chapter 4
Pharmaceutical Care Issues of Rheumatoid Arthritis Patients

Lilian M. Azzopardi, Louise Grech, and Marilyn Rogers

4.1 Introduction

Along the years, pharmacy as a profession has come a long way. It has grown from the traditional role of the pharmacist-compounder, preparing and dispensing extemporaneous preparations within community pharmacies, to the role of the pharmacist dispensing ready-made medicines within community pharmacies [1–6]. This move from product focus to patient focus brought to the forefront the pharmacist intervention as an advisor and coordinator of care. The profession has expanded also within the pharmaceutical industry where pharmacists contribute at various levels within the pharmaceutical industry ranging from research and development for innovative drugs, quality control to pharmacovigilance and pharmaceutical regulatory affairs personnel. The pharmacy profession has made major strides within the hospital setting with clinical pharmacists participating as the fulcrum of a multidisciplinary team and contributing to the decision-making for patient care. In this evolution of the pharmacy profession, the patient's well-being is the focus of pharmacist's activities in whichever setting they are practising, and this is what makes a pharmacist a unique player in the different settings.

L.M. Azzopardi, PhD (✉)
Department of Pharmacy, Faculty of Medicine and Surgery, Faculties of Pharmacies,
University of Malta, Msida, Malta
e-mail: lilian.m.azzopardi@um.edu.mt

L. Grech, PhD (✉)
Clinical Pharmacy Practice Unit, Department of Pharmacy, Mater Dei Hospital,
Msida, Malta

Department of Pharmacy, Faculty of Medicine and Surgery, University of Malta, Msida, Malta
e-mail: louise.grech@um.edu.mt

M. Rogers, MD, MRCP (UK) (✉)
Department of Medicine, Mater Dei Hospital, Msida, Malta
e-mail: marilynmifsud@yahoo.com

© Springer Science+Business Media Singapore 2016
L. Grech, A. Lau (eds.), *Pharmaceutical Care Issues of Patients
with Rheumatoid Arthritis*, DOI 10.1007/978-981-10-1421-5_4

The pharmacist, irrespective of whether working within the community, hospital or pharmaceutical industry setting, is a healthcare professional having the necessary clinical and pharmaceutical expertise who can provide advice and quality assurance within a multidisciplinary healthcare team involving the patient [7, 8]. The profession is patient centred and at the basis of the profession is the concept of pharmaceutical care. This chapter draws on clinical examples pertaining to pharmaceutical care issues of rheumatoid arthritis in order to illustrate the contribution of the pharmacist. It also describes the use of the RhMAT, an innovative tool that could be implemented within pharmaceutical care plans for rheumatoid arthritis.

4.2 Pharmaceutical Care: The Contribution of the Pharmacy Profession

The concept of 'pharmaceutical care', which can be defined as 'the responsible provision of drug therapy for the purpose of achieving definite outcomes that improve a patient's quality of life' was put forward in the 1990s by Professor Charles Hepler and Linda Strand [9]. The definition captures the salient aspects of the service provided by pharmacists, through which pharmacists aid in clinical decision-making to ensure specific therapeutic outcomes. In rheumatoid arthritis, the specific therapeutic outcomes constituting a comprehensive pharmaceutical care plan include the management of the condition; reduction and elimination of rheumatoid arthritis symptoms such as pain, morning stiffness and decreased mobility; slowing or possibly stopping disease progression; and preventing disease-related comorbidities associated with rheumatoid arthritis such as by ensuring coadministration of prophylactic treatment for rheumatoid arthritis patients at risk of developing osteoporosis. In order to achieve these therapeutic outcomes within pharmaceutical care models, pharmacists must work in liaison with other members of the healthcare team, including rheumatologists, nurses, physiotherapists, occupational therapists and podiatrists. This professional intercollaboration ensures an optimum pharmacotherapy plan which is tailor-made to each individual patient's requirements, subsequently improving or maintaining the patient's quality of life [10, 11].

The contribution of pharmacists within rheumatoid arthritis pharmaceutical care models stems from principles of 'treat to target', 'early referral' for appropriate pharmacotherapy and the safe use of individualised 'personalised' pharmacotherapy. The focus of pharmaceutical care processes is to identify pharmaceutical care issues and drug therapy problems and seek ways to resolve these issues through an individualised pharmaceutical care plan [12]. Several pharmaceutical care models within the field of rheumatoid arthritis have been the focus of research work. These highlight the positive impact of the pharmaceutical care service on improving the quality of service provided, decreasing financial constraints and improving the quality of life of rheumatoid arthritis patients [10, 13–20]. Pharmacists are in a central position in identifying pharmaceutical care issues and engaging in clinical decision-making within a pharmaceutical care model with the aim of ensuring optimum patient care and improvement in the quality of life of rheumatoid arthritis patients.

4.3 Categorisation of Pharmaceutical Care Issues in Rheumatoid Arthritis

In clinical practice, pharmacists providing pharmaceutical care sessions to rheumatoid arthritis patients identify pharmaceutical care issues. These pharmaceutical care issues can be classified as 'drug therapy problems' defined as 'undesirable events or risks experienced by the patient that involve or are suspected to involve drug therapy and which inhibit or delay the patient from achieving the desired goals of treatment' [21].

The drug therapy problems can be further subdivided into *actual* and *potential* drug therapy problems according to a classification implemented by Scottish pharmacists-researchers and colleagues, led by Professor Steve Hudson and Dr John McAnaw. Actual drug therapy problems are problems which are present at the time of the pharmaceutical care session and should be resolved immediately. Potential drug therapy problems are problems which are not yet present but which might arise in future and which could be avoided if timely action is taken. The aspect of potential drug therapy problems presents a role for the pharmacist as being proactive and pre-empting potential problems, thereby increasing and ensuring patient safety. This categorisation system is implemented in the rheumatology clinic at Mater Dei Hospital, Malta, and has been the subject of research work by one of the authors [18]. Figure 4.1 illustrates the drug therapy problems categorisation scheme.

4.3.1 Case Scenarios

A holistic approach needs to be adopted when screening for pharmaceutical care issues and drug therapy problems in rheumatoid arthritis patients who are known to have added comorbidities. This holistic approach forms part of the individualised and personalised pharmacotherapy plan, taking into consideration the specific requirements of each individual patient. A personalised approach offering the right treatment to the right patient according to their specific needs results in optimum use of medications within a safety index and a pharmacoeconomic aspect [22]. The identified drug therapy problems need to be appropriately documented and discussed with the respective clinician and the patient. Medication adherence, polypharmacy, drug interactions, prescription errors and lack of appropriate monitoring or lack of the patient's ability or willingness to attend for

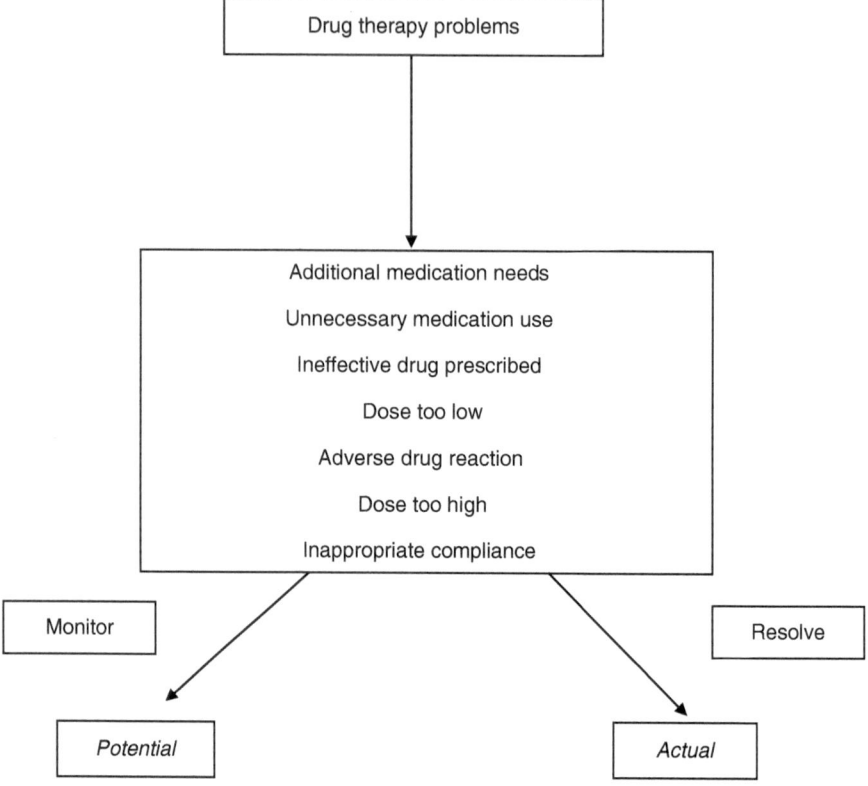

Fig. 4.1 Categorisation of drug therapy problems (Source: Drawn from McAnaw [77]. Adapted from Bayraktar [76] and from Azzopardi [75])

the requested blood and laboratory investigations could result in a number of drug therapy problems. Table 4.1 illustrates a few clinical case scenarios of various drug therapy problems.

4.3.2 Patient Monitoring Within Pharmaceutical Care Models

The synthetic DMARDs and the biologic DMARDs all require a certain amount of monitoring in order to ensure their safe use. The monitoring of DMARDs is generally related to the prevention of adverse reactions relating to bone marrow suppression such as pancytopenia, as well as liver impairment and renal impairment [23, 24]. Monitoring guidelines such as those issued by the British Society for Rheumatology help clinicians adhere to correct monitoring when using DMARDs [25]. In general, each hospital or trust will have local guidelines on monitoring of DMARDs. Table 4.2 summarises the monitoring required with DMARDs.

Table 4.1 Actual and potential drug therapy problems in clinical practice

Drug therapy problem	Actual or potential	Clinical examples
Additional medication	Actual	Addition of biologic DMARD to methotrexate 25 mg weekly in a patient who remains uncontrolled
	Potential	Use of calcium supplementation in a female patient who is at high risk of developing osteoporosis
Unnecessary medication	Actual	RA patient is well controlled on methotrexate and hydroxychloroquine but is still taking prednisolone 15 mg as prescribed at last visit when hydroxychloroquine was also added. Prednisolone is no longer required and can be stopped because the combination of the DMARDs should be enough
	Potential	Patient is on a proton pump inhibitor (PPI) in absence of any drugs which induce heartburn
Ineffective drug prescribed	Actual	Hydroxychloroquine which is a mild DMARD is prescribed in a patient with poor prognostic factors. There are no contraindications to methotrexate which should be prescribed instead
	Potential	A patient who is on methotrexate weekly and adalimumab 40 mg alternate weeks which was started approximately 6 weeks before complains that there are no signs of improvement. A treatment review in terms of the biologic drug may be required. The pharmacist could double check with the patient that the adalimumab is being correctly stored. Adalimumab being a biologic drug and protein in nature should be stored at a temperature between 2 and 8° Celsius. Inappropriate storage can lead to denaturing of the drug leading to ineffectiveness
Suboptimum dose prescribed	Actual	A patient is prescribed infliximab 3 mg/kg every 8 weeks, but the RA is not controlled. The dose prescribed is subsequently increased to 3 mg/kg every 6 weeks
	Potential	A patient's relative presents a prescription for methotrexate 2.5 mg weekly. According to previous pharmaceutical care profile of the patient, the dose should read 12.5 mg weekly
Adverse drug reactions	Actual	Nausea and vomiting in patients on methotrexate. One possible suggestion would be to change to the parenteral route
	Potential	Patient recently started on tocilizumab is noted to have an elevation in the lipid profile in comparison to baseline lipid profile. This elevation could be the result of tocilizumab. The patient however admits that there was a change in diet due to recent festivities. Further monitoring of the lipid profile is required
Dose too high	Actual	A patient presents a prescription of leflunomide 100 mg daily. The patient has been on leflunomide for the past 2 years. The correct dose should be 10–20 mg daily as this is the maintenance dose

(continued)

Table 4.1 (continued)

Drug therapy problem	Actual or potential	Clinical examples
	Potential	Patient presents a prescription for prednisolone 10 mg alternating with 5 mg daily. During discharge counselling, the pharmacist notes that the patient was under the impression that he was meant to take 10 mg in the morning and 5 mg in the evening every day
Inappropriate compliance	Actual	A patient is prescribed once weekly oral methotrexate and etanercept subcutaneous injection. The patient suffers from diabetes mellitus, ischaemic heart disease and epilepsy and has multiple other medications. The patient feels that etanercept is sufficient and confesses that she does not take the prescribed methotrexate dose
	Potential	A widower has been recently diagnosed with early dementia, and the patient is concerned that he will not be able to remember to take the weekly methotrexate. The patient is counselled on the use of medication aids such as alarms and marking the calendar and the use of pillbox which can be prepared by relatives or carers

Table 4.2 Monitoring required with respect to commonly prescribed DMARDs

DMARD	Prescreening	Routine
Methotrexate	Complete blood count, liver function tests, renal function tests, baseline chest X-Ray	Complete blood count, liver function tests, renal function tests
Sulphasalazine	Complete blood count, liver function tests, renal function tests	Complete blood count, liver function tests
Leflunomide	Complete blood count, liver function tests, renal function tests, blood pressure measured on 2 occasions at least 2 weeks apart, baseline body weight	Complete blood count, liver function tests, regular blood pressure and body weight
Hydroxychloroquine	Liver function tests, renal function tests, visual acuity	Annual ophthalmic review
Azathioprine	Complete blood count, liver function tests, renal function tests	Complete blood count, liver function tests, renal function tests
Ciclosporin	Complete blood count, liver function tests, lipid profile and renal function tests with serum creatinine and blood pressure being checked twice, 2 weeks apart	Complete blood count, liver function tests, renal function tests and regular blood pressure monitoring

Monitoring in relation to biologic DMARDs is more or less the same for all the biologic DMARDs. Prescreening required for patients who are to be started on any biologic DMARD includes hepatitis B and C tests, screening for HIV and screening for tuberculosis. Biologic DMARDs are highly immunosuppressive drugs, and potentially serious infections such as hepatitis B, hepatitis C, HIV and untreated tuberculosis can lead to life-threatening situations [26, 27]. Ensuring appropriate prescreening is one of the contributions of the pharmacist towards safe use of biologic DMARDs. In addition, tocilizumab requires regular lipid and liver tests, whereas anakinra necessitates the regular monitoring of complete blood count in order identify neutropenia since treatment with anakinra has been commonly associated with neutropenia. There are no guidelines which dictate the regular monitoring of complete blood count, renal function and liver function in patients on biologic DMARDs, but in practice clinicians do order regular blood investigations especially since most patients are on concomitant DMARD treatment such as methotrexate.

The contribution of the pharmacist within this aspect lies in ensuring correct and timely monitoring as per guidelines and explaining the importance of adherence to the required monitoring [28]. Two real case scenarios are described to highlight the important role of the pharmacist in enhancing appropriate patient monitoring, thus safeguarding the patients' health.

4.3.2.1 Real Case Scenario 1

Mr JX is a 53-year-old gentleman who has been suffering from rheumatoid arthritis for the past 20 years. He is currently on regular methotrexate 25 mg weekly, folic acid 10 mg weekly and infliximab administered at a dose of 5 mg/kg every 8 weeks. The patient presents to the Day Unit for his scheduled infliximab. Prior to the drug administration, the clinical pharmacist checks his blood profile and notes that the patient is not booked for further complete blood counts and renal and liver function tests and he does not have a scheduled appointment with the rheumatologist. This is confirmed with the patient who states that he has no further appointments with the rheumatologist nor appointments for bloods tests. The pharmacist alerts the rheumatologist to book the necessary appointments.

4.3.2.2 Real Case Scenario 2

Mrs RM is a 30-year-old lady diagnosed 2 years ago with rheumatoid arthritis and is on sulphasalazine 1 g three times daily. The lady presents to pick up her medication, and the pharmacist notes that Mrs RM has not been to the phlebotomy clinic for her scheduled blood investigations and subsequently there are no results for the complete blood count and renal and liver function tests. This is not the first time this has happened over the past year, and the patient admits that ever since getting a promotion, her life has become more hectic, and attending for blood investigations is a waste of time. The pharmacist discusses the issue with the patient and explains that compliance to blood investigations ordered by the clinician ensures safe use of sulphasalazine.

4.4   The RhMAT as an Innovative Tool
Within Pharmaceutical Care Models

The role of the pharmacist in identifying pharmaceutical care issues is established. But how can pharmacists further develop the pharmaceutical care service to a higher level and integrate higher standards of care delivered to rheumatoid arthritis patients? What tools are required to support pharmacists to offer the best service, ensuring quality of care? The RhMAT, Rheumatoid Arthritis Medication Assessment Tool, is a novel tool that integrates quality of care and pharmaceutical care issues within the pharmaceutical care models. It is a tool which can be used by pharmacists practising with rheumatoid arthritis patients to further sustain a stronger service.

The concept of medication assessment tools introduced by the University of Strathclyde researchers is a way forward in the design and implementation of pharmaceutical care models [29]. Medication assessment tools are evidence-based instruments with the aim of evaluating, prescribing and monitoring adherence to established guidelines in specific conditions. Validated medication assessment tools have been developed for a number of chronic conditions including heart failure and coronary artery disease, diabetes mellitus, pain management in cancer patients and asthma [30–34]. Medication assessment tools offer a systematic approach in identifying pharmaceutical care issues and also identifying gaps to established guidelines which can be resolved within a multidisciplinary team.

The major clinical contributions of the RhMAT are twofold: namely, its ability to capture the degree of adherence of each individual patient's pharmacotherapy plan to evidence-based guidelines and its ability to identify the actual gaps which lead to the degree of non-adherence towards evidence-based guidelines. The RhMAT can be used in a clinical practice setting within a pharmaceutical care model to capture pharmaceutical care issues and identify and close pharmacotherapy gaps, thereby improving the quality of care service offered to patients, thus enhancing patients' safety and quality of life [35].

4.4.1   Design and In-Practice Application of the RhMAT

The RhMAT consists of criteria based on latest evidence-based guidelines, recommendations and standards on rheumatoid arthritis and its management as set out by the leading experts in the field, namely, the American College of Rheumatology (ACR), the European League against Rheumatism (EULAR), the British Society for Rheumatology (BSR) and the National Institute for Health and Care Excellence (NICE). The summary of product characteristics for each drug included in the RhMAT is used as reference for criteria related to drug pharmacological properties such as contraindications and counselling [35].

A general instructions sheet for the RhMAT is available as a user reference guide. The instructions, which define the outcome that can be chosen for each criterion listed, help promote uniformity in clinical settings where the tool is used by different raters.

The RhMAT is designed in the form of a table allowing the pharmacist to be able to easily document the necessary response in the least possible time-consuming manner. The RhMAT consists of 11 separate sections dealing with:

i. Diagnosis of rheumatoid arthritis
ii. Use of analgesics and nonsteroidal anti-inflammatory drugs
iii. Use of methotrexate
iv. Use of sulphasalazine
v. Use of hydroxychloroquine
vi. Use of leflunomide
vii. Use of sodium aurothiomalate parenteral preparation
viii. General screening for biological therapies
ix. Use of biological therapies
x. Use of glucocorticoids
xi. Remission cases

Each criterion is judged for applicability and adherence in practice. If the criterion is applicable, a 'Yes' answer is required. If the criterion is not met, then the response would be 'No'. If the 'No' response is justified according to a logistic reason, then it is a justified No (No$_J$) and the justification is given in the comments section. If the 'No' is unjustified, then the (No$_{UJ}$) should be marked. In the case of the criterion adherence which cannot be determined due to incomplete data which cannot be collected through the patient's medical case notes and neither through the patient's interview, then the response to the criterion should be marked as insufficient data (ID) [35]. Table 4.3 illustrates an extract from the RhMAT.

The RhMAT incorporates a mathematical equation which yields the adherence rate to the criteria included in the tool. Adherence rate to the RhMAT is calculated as the sum of the 'Yes' responses expressed as a percentage of the total number of applicable cases whereby the applicable cases constitute the number of 'Yes' responses, the 'No unjustified' (No$_{uj}$) responses and the 'insufficient data' (ID) responses:

$$\text{Adherence} = \frac{\sum(\text{Yes})}{\sum(\text{Yes} + \text{NO}_{uj} + \text{ID})} \times 100$$

The total adherence rate to the RhMAT incorporating all the 11 sections can be calculated. The adherence rate to each of the separate individual applicable sections depending on the drugs prescribed for individual patients can also be calculated. Therefore, if a patient is on methotrexate and sulphasalazine, the pharmacist can calculate the total RhMAT adherence rate as well as the adherence rate for the individual sections pertaining to methotrexate and sulphasalazine separately. The average time taken to complete the RhMAT in an outpatient clinic setting is 15 min.

Table 4.3 RhMAT extract: sections on use of methotrexate and biologics

	N/A	Yes	NoJ	No$_{UJ}$	ID	Pharmacist's comments
Methotrexate						
1. Used as a first-line DMARD in absence of contraindications	❏	❏	❏	❏	❏	
2. Pretreatment screening including chest X-ray, CBC, ESR, CRP, LFTs, renal profile, in accordance with local protocol	❏	❏	❏	❏	❏	
3. Regular monitoring according to monitoring protocol schedule including mouth ulcers, nausea and vomiting, dyspnoea	❏	❏	❏	❏	❏	
4. Contraindications, namely, pregnancy, breastfeeding, active local or systemic infection, bone marrow suppression excluded	❏	❏	❏	❏	❏	
5. The patient has been prescribed methotrexate at dose that is unambiguously expressed as a ONCE a WEEK administration	❏	❏	❏	❏	❏	
6. The patient has been counselled and information leaflet given	❏	❏	❏	❏	❏	
7. Issues of family planning and breast feeding have been explained to the patient	❏	❏	❏	❏	❏	
8. Patient is coprescribed folic acid 10 mg weekly	❏	❏	❏	❏	❏	
General screening for biologic therapy						
1. Patient satisfies EULAR recommendation criteria for starting biological therapy	❏	❏	❏	❏	❏	
2. Pretreatment screening including screening for mycobacterial infections (Quantiferon test), hepatitis B, hepatitis C and HIV in accordance with local protocol has been carried out	❏	❏	❏	❏	❏	
3. Patient has been counselled about the treatment, namely, side effects, family planning, live vaccines, malignancy	❏	❏	❏	❏	❏	
4. Routine follow-up monitoring including DAS examination and blood investigations	❏	❏	❏	❏	❏	

4.5 Quality-of-Life Tools Within Pharmaceutical Care Models

In everyday life, rheumatoid arthritis can have an impact on various physical and psychological domains of the patients, ranging from moods and emotions, social life, hobbies, activities of daily living, and personal and social relationships. Rheumatoid arthritis affects patients' quality of life [36–42].

Quality-of-life tools gather information from the patients' perspective about the impact the disease is having on their day-to-day living and to what extent the condition is interfering with the patients' lifestyle. Quality-of-life tools are instrumental in evaluating the response of patients to pharmacotherapy prescribed in the management of chronic conditions such as rheumatoid arthritis. Appropriate changes in pharmacotherapy may affect a patient's quality of life in a positive or negative manner, leading to health-related quality-of-life outcomes. Pharmacists can make use of quality-of-life tools in order to assess and adjust pharmacotherapy accordingly, with the aim of improving health-related quality-of-life outcomes. Such quality-of-life tools can be used as adjuvant tools to the RhMAT within pharmaceutical care models [18, 43].

4.5.1   Generic and Specific Health-Related Quality-of-Life Tools

There are two main approaches to assess health-related quality of life, namely, using disease-specific tools or generic (general) tools.

Specific rheumatoid arthritis health-related quality-of-life instruments are specific to rheumatoid arthritis based on the extent of functional disability caused by the condition. These tools are more sensitive to changes characteristic to the progression of rheumatoid arthritis [44].

There are various rheumatoid arthritis-specific health-related questionnaires including:

* Health Assessment Questionnaire (HAQ) [45]
* Arthritis Impact Measurement Scales (AIMS) [46]
* McMaster Toronto Arthritis Patient Preference Disability Questionnaire (MACTAR) [47]
* Functional Status Index (FSI) [48]
* Toronto Functional Capacity Questionnaire (TFCQ) [49]

The Health Assessment Questionnaire is however the most widely used due to its practicality within a clinical setting, validity and reliability [50–53]. The Health Assessment Questionnaire (HAQ) targets specifically the activities of daily living. The domains of the Health Assessment Questionnaire consist of eight categories, namely, dressing, arising, eating, walking, hygiene, reaching, gripping and running errands. Each category has two to three questions aimed to quantify the difficulties in performing daily activities. The patient is given a choice of four response options on a Likert scale ranging from 'without any difficulty' score 1, 'with some difficulty' score 2, 'with much difficulty' score 3 and 'unable to do' score 4. The maximum score for each question in each of the eight categories of the HAQ is taken to represent the score for that category. The maximum scores of each of the eight categories are added up and subsequently divided by 8 (the total number of the categories) to give a mean HAQ score ranging between 0 and 3 [45, 50, 51]. Clinically, a mean score of 0 indicates *no difficulty*, a score of 1 indicates *some difficulty*, a score of 2 indicates *much difficulty or assistance needed*, and a score of 3 indicates *unable to perform*. The lower the score, the better the quality of life. A HAQ score greater than or equal to 1.5 indicates limitation in performing activities of daily living and possibly the need to review pharmacotherapy with the aim of optimising drug therapy.

In contrast to disease-specific health-related quality-of-life tools, generic health-related questionnaires are designed to assess a complete range of dimensions which apply to a variety of health states, conditions and diseases. These are therefore not restricted and not specific to particular conditions offering a holistic approach to patients who very often have comorbidities. Generic health-related tools can also be used to provide data which allows comparison between a variety of different diseases. Examples of generic health-related quality-of-life instruments include:

- The Sickness Impact Profile (SIP) [54]
- Quality of Well-Being Index (QWB) [55]
- Nottingham Health Profile (NHP) [56]
- Medical Outcomes Study Short Form 36 (SF36) [57]

The Medical Outcomes Study Short Form 36 (SF36) is the most widely generic tool used in rheumatology conditions including rheumatoid arthritis. The SF36 consists of one multi-item scale which assesses eight health concepts or domains:

1. Limitations in physical activities due to health problems
2. Limitations in social activities due to physical or emotional problems
3. Limitations in usual role activities due to physical health problems
4. Effect of body pain
5. General mental health including extent of psychological distress and well-being
6. Limitations in usual role activities due to emotional problems
7. Vitality
8. General health perceptions

The SF36 provides individual scoring for the eight subscales and takes approximately 10 min to complete [57]. The Health Assessment Questionnaire and the Medical Outcomes Study Short Form 36 questionnaire are the health-related quality-of-life tools mostly quoted in studies relating to rheumatoid arthritis [58–64].

4.6   Medication Adherence as Part of Pharmaceutical Care Models

Medication adherence encompasses a relationship between the prescriber and the willingness of the patient to adhere to the prescribed plan which has been specifically designed together with the patient to accommodate the patient's lifestyle. It is useless prescribing and ensuring that the best practice pharmacotherapy is prescribed according to the latest evidence-based guidelines to meet each individual patient needs without taking into consideration the patient's perception. In practice, it is futile to prescribe subcutaneous biologic DMARDs, which are costly, to patients who are unwilling and do not agree on taking such treatment. It is also useless prescribing methotrexate to patients who refuse to take methotrexate because of fear of its potential side effects. Therefore, the possibility of patient non-adherence with prescribed pharmacotherapy which could result due to the patient's own characteristics, perceptions, beliefs and concerns and sometimes cultural issues needs to be taken into consideration when prescribing [65–67].

The contribution of the pharmacist towards improving patients' medication adherence is of utmost importance [68]. The responsibility of the pharmacist lies in two aspects, namely, through patient education and through the ability and responsibility of the pharmacist to understand and listen to the concerns voiced by patients with respect to their prescribed pharmacotherapy. Firstly, patient education and empowerment are of utmost importance and form an integral part of pharmaceutical care sessions. It is the responsibility of the pharmacist, as the drug expert, who is also in a coordinating position within the multidisciplinary team, to carry out patient counselling on pharmacotherapy. Patients need to be aware and to fully understand why each drug is being prescribed, thereby increasing the patients' confidence in the necessity of the pharmacotherapy being used to reduce or eliminate disease progression which will otherwise lead to decreased quality of life. Secondly, and equally important is that pharmacists need to listen to the patients' concerns and fears about their prescribed medications. Studies have shown that patient education together with prescribers' and pharmacists' understanding of patients' concerns about the medications prescribed further improves patients' adherence in long-term chronic conditions such as rheumatoid arthritis. Medication adherence in turn improves patients' quality of life and reduces waste and financial constrains in relation to unused medication [69–74].

Effective management of rheumatoid arthritis and avoidance of progression of the condition results from both the appropriate evidence-based prescribing of pharmacotherapy as well as patients' adherence to the pharmacotherapy prescribed.

Take Home Messages
- Pharmacists are the sole healthcare professionals able to provide a pharmaceutical care service.
- The RhMAT is a novel medication assessment tool specifically designed for rheumatoid arthritis.
- The RhMAT aids pharmacists to capture the degree of adherence of the pharmacotherapy prescribed for each patient in relation to the latest evidence-based guidelines.
- The RhMAT also aids pharmacists to identify pharmacotherapy gaps which result in pharmaceutical care issues.
- Identification of pharmaceutical care issues allows the pharmacist to work in close collaboration with rheumatologists in order to suggest the best possible pharmacotherapy tailor-made to each individual patient's needs sustaining the contribution of the pharmacist as an essential healthcare provider in clinical decision-making.
- The use of health-related quality-of-life tools within pharmaceutical care models should be encouraged to aid in providing a holistic approach to care.
- As part of the pharmaceutical care model, pharmacists are key healthcare professionals able to offer counselling and patient education on medications, thereby increasing medication adherence.
- Pharmaceutical care service provision results in improved patient care, quality of life, reduction in medication waste and subsequently reduction in financial constraints.

References

1. Pearson GJ (2007) Evolution in the practice of pharmacy – not a revolution! CMAJ 176(9):1295–1296
2. Franchino DC (2010) Redefining the pharmacist's role. Am J Health-Syst Pharm 67:178
3. Woodward B (2011) Implementing practice model change: opportunities and challenges in a changing environment. Am J Health-Syst Pharm 68:1099–1100
4. Zellmer WA (2012) The future of health-system pharmacy: opportunities and challenges in practice model change. Ann Pharmacother 46(4):S41–S45
5. Weber RJ, Stevenson JG, White SJ (2013) Measuring change in health-system pharmacy over 50 years: reflecting on the mirror, Part II. Hosp Pharm 48(11):966–969
6. Weber RJ, Stevenson JG, White SJ (2014) Measuring change in health-system pharmacy over 50 years: reflecting on the mirror, Part II. Hosp Pharm 49(1):97–100
7. Hudson S, McAnaw JJ, Johnson BJ (2007) The changing roles of pharmacists in society. Int e-J Med Educ 1:22–34
8. Chisholm-Burns MA, Kim Lee J, Spivey CA, Slack M, Herrier RN, Hall-Lipsy E et al (2010) US pharmacists' effect as team members on patient care: systematic review and meta-analyses. Med Care 48(10):923–933
9. Hepler CD, Strand LM (1990) Opportunities and responsibilities in pharmaceutical care. Am J Hosp Pharm 47(3):533–543
10. Hudson S, Bayraktar A, McAnaw J (2003) Pharmaceutical care issues in the management of rheumatoid arthritis. Int J Adv Rheumatol 1(3):97–103
11. Flick C, Farrell J (2013) The role of the pharmacist in the management of rheumatic disease. The Rheumatologist 1–4
12. Tulip S, Campbell D (2001) Evaluating pharmaceutical care in hospitals. Hosp Pharm 8:275–279
13. Green C (2003) Pharmaceutical care in rheumatoid arthritis. Hosp Pharm Europe 11
14. O'Hare R, Muir A, Chapman S, Watson A, Hudson SA (2001) Identification of the pharmaceutical care issues of rheumatoid arthritis patients in secondary care. Pharm World Sci 23(5):183–184
15. Bayraktar A, Hudson S, Watson S, Fraser A (2000) Pharmaceutical care: arthritis. Pharm J 274:57–68
16. Griscti S, Serracino Inglott A, Zarb Adami M, Azzopardi LM, Mallia C, Azzopardi L et al (2010) Management of rheumatoid arthritis. Hosp Pharm Europe 49:20–21
17. Barlow JF, Faris RJ, Wang W, Verbrugge RR, Garavaglia SB, Aubert RE (2012) Impact of speciality pharmacy on treatment costs for rheumatoid arthritis. Am J Pharm Benefits 4:SP49–SP56
18. Grech L, Coleiro B, Borg A, Serracino Inglott A, Azzopardi LM (2013) Evaluation of the pharmaceutical care service offered to rheumatoid arthritis patients within an ambulatory setting. Am J Pharm Health Res 1(7):78–86
19. Bornstein C, Craig M, Tin D (2014) The pharmacological management of rheumatoid arthritis with traditional and biologic disease modifying anti-rheumatic drugs. Practice guidelines for pharmacists. Can Pharm J 147(2):97–109
20. Gong L, Wooley MC, Glasser CE, Bumpass JB, Sekab J, Skirvin JA (2014) Rheumatoid arthritis: aggressive new treatment guidelines. US Pharmacist 2014;39(11)(Speciality & Oncology suppl):3–7
21. Cipolle RJ, Strand LM, Morley PC, Frakes M (2004) Pharmaceutical Care Practice; the clinician's guide. McGraw Hill, New York, pp 78–79, 165
22. Karsden MA, Bay-Jensen AC, Henriksen K, Christiansen C, Genant HK, Chamberlain C et al (2014) Rheumatoid arthritis: a case for personalised health care? Arthritis Care Res 66(9):1273–1280
23. Highton J, Harrison A, Grainger R (2008) Rheumatoid arthritis – monitoring of DMARDs. Best Pract J 17:22–32

24. Ruderman EM (2012) Overview of safety of non-biologic and biologic DMARDs. Rheumatology 51(Suppl 6):vi37–vi43
25. Chakravarty K, McDonald H, Pullar T, Taggart A, Chalmers R, Oliver S et al (2008) BSR/BHPR guideline for disease modifying anti-rheumatic drug (DMARD) therapy in consultation with the British Association of Dermatologists. Rheumatology 47(6):924–925
26. Ding T, Ledingham J, Luqmani R, Westlake S, Hyrich K, Lunt M et al (2010) BSR and BHPR rheumatoid arthritis guidelines on safety of anti-TNF therapies. Rheumatology 49:2217–2219
27. The British Society for Rheumatology (2005) Update on the British Society for Rheumatology guidelines for prescribing TNF-alfa blockers in adults with rheumatoid arthritis (update of previous guidelines of April 2001). Rheumatology 44:157–163
28. Chew LC, Yee SL (2013) The Rheumatology Monitoring Clinic in Singapore – a novel advanced practice nurse/pharmacist-led clinic. Proc Singapore Healthcare 22(1):48–55
29. McAnaw J, Hudson S, McGlynn S (2003) Development of an evidence-based medication assessment tools to demonstrate the quality of drug therapy use in patients with heart failure. Int J Pharm Pract 11:R17
30. Hakonsen GD, Strelec P, Campbell D, Hudson S, Loennechen T (2009) Adherence to medication guideline criteria in pain management. J Pain Symptom Manage 37(6):1006–1018
31. Diab M, Johnson J, Hudson S (2013) Adherence to clinical guidelines in management of diabetes and prevention of cardiovascular disease in Qatar. Int J Clin Pharm 35(1):101–112
32. Dreischulte T, Johnson J, McAnaw J, Geurts M, de Gier H, Hudson S (2013) Medication assessment tool to detect care issues from routine data: a pilot study in primary care. Int J Clin Pharm 35(6):1063–1074
33. Garcia B, Smabrekke L, Trovik T, Giverhaug T (2013) Application of the MAT-CHDSP to assess guideline adherence and therapy goal achievement in secondary prevention of coronary heart disease after percutaneous coronary intervention. Eur J Clin Pharmacol 69(3):703–709
34. Liu P, Chen HY, Johnson J, Lin YM (2013) A medication assessment tool to evaluate adherence to medication guideline in asthmatic children. Int J Clin Pharm 35(2):289–295
35. Grech L, Ferrito V, Serracino Inglott A, Azzopardi LM (2016) Development of the RhMAT, as medication tool specifically designed for rheumatoid arthritis management. J Pharm Health Serv Res 7(1):89–92
36. Daul P, Grisanti J (2009) Monitoring response to therapy in rheumatoid arthritis. Bull NHU Hosp Jt Dis 67(2):236–242
37. Walker JG, Littlejohn GO (2007) Measuring quality of life in rheumatic conditions. Clin Rheumatol 26:671–673
38. Tugwell P, Idzerda L, Wells GA (2008) Generic quality of life assessment in rheumatoid arthritis. Am J Manag Care 14(4):234
39. Laas K, Roine R, Rasanen P, Sintonen H, Leirisalo-Repo M, HUS QoL Study Group (2009) Health-related quality of life in patients with common rheumatic diseases referred to a university clinic. Rheumatol Int 29(3):267–273
40. Chung KC, Pushman AG (2011) Current concepts in the management of the rheumatoid hand. J Hand Surg Am 36(4):736–747
41. Geryk LL, Carpenter DM, Blalock SJ, De Vellis RF, Jordan JM (2015) The impact of co-morbidity on health-related quality of life in rheumatoid arthritis and osteoarthritis patients. Clin Exp Rheumatol 33(3):366–374
42. Matcham F, Scott IC, Rayner L, Hotopf M, Kingsley GH, Norton S et al (2014) The impact of rheumatoid arthritis on quality of life assessed using the SF36: a systematic review and meta-analysis. Semin Arthritis Rheum 44(2):123–130
43. Kheir NM, van Mil JW, Shaw JP, Sheridan JL (2004) Health-related quality of life measurement in pharmaceutical care. Targeting an outcome that matters. Pharm World Sci 26(3):125–128
44. Wells GA, Russell AS, Haraoui B, Bissonnette R, Ware CF (2011) Validity of quality of life measurement tools: from generic to disease specific. J Rheumatol 88:2–6

45. Fries JF, Spitz P, Kraines RG, Holman HR (1980) Measurement of patient outcome in arthritis. Arthritis Rheum 23:137–145
46. Meenan RF, Gertman PM, Mason JH (1980) Measuring health status in arthritis: the Arthritis Impact Measurement Scales. Arthritis Rheum 23:146–152
47. Tugwell P, Bombadier C, Buchanan WW, Goldsmith CH, Grace E (1987) The MACTAR Questionnaire – an individualized functional priority approach for assessing improvement in physical disability in clinical trials in rheumatoid arthritis. J Rheumatol 14:446–451
48. Jette AM (1987) The functional status index: reliability and validity of a self-report functional disability measure. J Rheumatol Suppl 15:15–21
49. Helewa A, Goldsmith CH, Smyth HA (1982) Independent measurement of functional capacity in rheumatoid arthritis. J Rheumatol 9:794–797
50. Bruce B, Fries JF (2003) The Stanford Health Assessment Questionnaire: dimensions and practical applications. Health Qual Life Outcomes 1:20
51. Bruce B, Fries JF (2005) The Health Assessment Questionnaire. Clin Exp Rheumatol 23(S39):S14–S18
52. Russell A (2008) Quality of life assessment in rheumatoid arthritis. Pharmacoeconomics 26(10):831–846
53. Maska L, Anderson J, Michaud K (2011) Measures of functional status and quality of life in rheumatoid arthritis. Arthritis Care Res 63(S11):S4–S13
54. Gilson BS, Gilson JS, Bergner M, Bobbitt RA, Kressel S, Pollard WE et al (1975) The Sickness Impact Profile: development of an outcome measure of health care. AJPH 65(12):1304–1310
55. Balaban DJ, Sagi PC, Goldfard NL, Nettler S (1986) Weights for scoring the quality of well being (QWB) instrument among rheumatoid arthritis: a comparison to general population weights. Med Care 24:973–980
56. McDowell IM, Martini CJM, Waugh W (1978) A method for self-assessment of disability before and after hip replacement operations. BMJ 2:857–859
57. Ware JE Jr, Sherbourne CD (1992) The MOS 36 item short form health survey (SF36). A conceptual framework and item selection. Med Care 30:473–483
58. Birrell FN, Hassell AB, Jones PW, Dawes PT (2000) How does the Short Form 36 health questionnaire (SF36) in rheumatoid arthritis (RA) relate to RA outcome measures and SF36 population values? A cross-sectional study. Clin Rheumatol 19(3):195–199
59. Kosinski M, Kujawski SC, Martin R, Wanke LA, Buatti MC, Ware JE Jr et al (2002) Health-related quality of life in early rheumatoid arthritis: impact of disease and treatment response. Am J Manag Care 8(3):231–240
60. Corbacho MI, Dapueto JJ (2010) Assessing the functional status and quality of life of patients with rheumatoid arthritis. Rev Bras Rheumatol 50(1):31–34
61. Picchianti-Diamanti A, Germano V, Ferlito C, Migliore A, D'Amelio R, Laganà B (2010) Health-related quality of life and disability in patients with rheumatoid, early rheumatoid and early psoriatic arthritis treated with etanercept. Qual Life Res 19(6):821–826
62. Genovese MC, Han C, Keystone EC, Hsia EC, Buchanan J, Gathany T et al (2012) Effect of golimumab on patient-reported outcomes in rheumatoid arthritis:results from the GO-FORWARD study. J Rheumatol 39(6):1185–1191
63. Strand V, Rentz AM, Cifaldi MA, Chen N, Roy S, Revicki D (2012) Health-related quality of life outcomes of adalimumab for patients with early rheumatoid arthritis: results from a randomised multicentre study. J Rheumatol 39(1):63–72
64. Bae SC, Gun SC, Mok CC, Khandker R, Nab HW, Koenig AS et al (2013) Improved health outcomes with etanercept versus DMARD therapy in an Asian population with established rheumatoid arthritis. BMC Musculoskelet Disord 14(13)
65. Salt E, Frazier SK (2011) Predictors of medication adherence in patients with rheumatoid arthritis. Drug Dev Res 72(8):756–763
66. Horne R, Chapman SCE, Parham R, Freemantle N, Forbes A (2013) Understanding patients' adherence-related beliefs about medicines prescribed for long-term conditions: a meta-analytic review of the necessity concerns framework. PLoS One 8(12):1–24

67. Hugtenburg J, Timmers L, Elders PJM, Vervloet M, van Dijk L (2013) Definitions, variants and causes of non-adherence with medications: a challenge for tailored interventions. Patient Prefer Adherence 7:675–682
68. Albrecht S (2011) The pharmacist's role in medication adherence. US Pharm 36(5):45–48
69. de Achaval S, Suarez-Almazor ME (2010) Treatment adherence to disease modifying anti-rheumatic drugs in patients with rheumatoid arthritis and systemic lupus erythematosus. Int J Clin Rheumatol 5(3):313–326
70. Hill J, Bird H, Johnson S (2001) Effect of patient education on adherence to drug treatment for rheumatoid arthritis: a randomised controlled trial. Ann Rheum Dis 60:869–875
71. De Thurah A, Norgaard M, Harder I, Stengaard-Pedersen K (2010) Compliance with methotrexate treatment in patients with rheumatoid arthritis: influence of patients' beliefs about medicine. A prospective cohort study. Rheumatol Int 30(11):1441–1448
72. van den Bemt BJ, Zwikker HE, van den Ende CH (2012) Medication adherence in patients with rheumatoid arthritis: a critical appraisal of the existing literature. Expert Rev Clin Immunol 8(4):337–351
73. Gadallah MA, Boulos DN, Gebrel A, Dewedar S, Morisky DE (2015) Assessment of rheumatoid arthritis patients' adherence to treatment. Am J Med Sci 349(2):151–156
74. Morgan C, McBeth J, Cordingley L, Watson K, Hyrich KL, Symmons DP et al (2015) The influence of behavioural and psychological factors on medication adherence over time in rheumatoid arthritis patients: a study in the biologics era. Rheumatology 54(10):1780–1791
75. McAnaw JJ (2003) Development of novel approaches to demonstrate the quality of drug therapy use. Dissertation. University of Strathclyde, Glasgow
76. Bayraktar A (2003) The provision of pharmaceutical care in a system for the use of methotrexate in the treatment of patients with rheumatoid arthritis. Dissertation. University of Strathclyde, Glasgow
77. Azzopardi L (2007) Developing a pharmaceutical care plan for patients with Rheumatoid Arthritis. MPhil thesis. Department of Pharmaceutical Sciences. University of Strathclyde, Glasgow

Chapter 5
Transitional Care: Caring Across the Interface

Karen Farrugia and Margarida Caramona

5.1 Introduction

It is no surprise and no news that patients experience problems and unwanted hassle when they move across different care settings such as from the primary to secondary care settings, and vice versa. Movement of patients across the healthcare interface may not be completely smooth-running.

The problem mainly stems from lack of communication which very often results from logistic issues rather than the unwanted desire of healthcare professionals at different setups to communicate with each other [1–3].

Healthcare professionals and policymakers are aware of this fallacy and aim to provide a seamless care scenario where patients move across care settings with the least possible problems, least potential risk for medication errors and if possible without unwanted patient harm [4–8]. This chapter discusses the movement of rheumatoid arthritis patients across primary and secondary care settings, underlining the required collaboration between the community pharmacy and the hospital pharmacy.

K. Farrugia, BPharm (Hons) (Melit) (✉)
Chemimart Group of Pharmacies, Msida, Malta
e-mail: karfarrugia@gmail.com

M. Caramona, PhD (✉)
Faculty of Pharmacy, European Association of Faculties of Pharmacies, University of Coimbra, Coimbra, Portugal
e-mail: magui@ff.uc.pt

© Springer Science+Business Media Singapore 2016
L. Grech, A. Lau (eds.), *Pharmaceutical Care Issues of Patients with Rheumatoid Arthritis*, DOI 10.1007/978-981-10-1421-5_5

5.2   The Hospital Pharmacist and the Community Pharmacist: Bridging the Gap

Pharmacists play an important role in medication reconciliation during transitional care to reduce medication errors and subsequent consequences [9–14]. In secondary care, medicine reconciliation is carried out by hospital pharmacists on admission and on discharge. On admission to hospital, medicine reconciliation is of utmost importance to rule out any potentially existing medication discrepancies. Medication reconciliation on admission provides the secondary care team with an accurate list of medications taken by the patients whilst in the primary care setting and at home [15–19].

Medication reconciliation on discharge forms an important part of the pharmaceutical care plan which aims to ensure continuity of care across the two interfaces [20–27]. Medication reconciliation on discharge is more complex than medication reconciliation on admission. On discharge, the pharmacist needs to ensure that the list of medications against which patients are being discharged is comprehensive. The discharge medications will include medications with which the patients presented to the hospital and which were not changed, those medications which were added on whilst in hospital and which need to be continued whilst at home and those medications, such as a course of prednisolone, which were started whilst in hospital but which need to be tapered down whilst the patient is at home. Discharge counselling is closely linked with medication reconciliation. On discharge, pharmacists provide discharge counselling to the patients educating them on the appropriate use and administration of medications such as frequency of administration, drug-food interactions, what side effects to expect and how to manage them amongst other aspects [28, 29]. Hospital pharmacists are the last point of contact most patients would encounter prior to being discharged back to the primary care setting and in the community setting.

Once in the primary and community setting, the community pharmacists become the first port of call for patients who might have queries, concerns or doubts about their medication. Despite appropriate counselling from the hospital pharmacists, patients may still be confused over their new medications or which medications need to be stopped or dose reduced after some time from discharge. Medicine reconciliation by community pharmacists at this stage confirms that patients understand and can follow the pharmacotherapy plan prescribed by the secondary care team thereby ensuring continuity of care [30, 31]. Furthermore community pharmacists are the healthcare professionals whom patients within the community and primary care setting are most likely to frequently visit. Very often, over time, a relationship of trust, confidence and friendship is built between the community pharmacists and their regular patients putting community pharmacists at the forefront of pharmaceutical care and chronic disease management within a community setting [32–40].

5.3 The Community Pharmacist's Contribution to Rheumatoid Arthritis Patients

Rheumatoid arthritis patients are followed up to an extent, through the out-patient setting and very rarely are admitted to hospital as in-patients for treatment of the condition itself. Rheumatoid arthritis can be considered as a chronic condition which is mainly managed through an out-patient setting. Community pharmacists who are dispensing the prescribed rheumatoid arthritis pharmacotherapy are ideally placed to design and implement individualised pharmaceutical care plans, subsequently identifying pharmaceutical care issues and drug therapy problems as they might arise. The pharmaceutical care model presented and discussed in Chap. 4 can be implemented by community pharmacists for rheumatoid arthritis patients whilst collaborating with pharmacists from the rheumatology hospital setting [41].

There are several ways in which community pharmacists can contribute towards optimum management and care of rheumatoid arthritis patients. Community pharmacists can capture patients showing early signs and symptoms indicative of rheumatoid arthritis subsequently referring the patients to clinicians for timely appropriate pharmacotherapy.

Whilst dispensing medications to the rheumatoid arthritis patients, the community pharmacists re-enforce patient counselling on the appropriate use and correct dosage regimen. They are also in an ideal situation to identify and prevent drug-drug interactions which can arise from time to time, such as the interaction between methotrexate and the antibiotic cotrimoxazole which could be prescribed to patients by clinicians who are unaware of the patients' use of methotrexate. Furthermore community pharmacists play an essential role in identifying and managing side effects in relation to pharmacotherapy used in rheumatoid arthritis. The community pharmacists can assess medication adherence and identify patients who fail to refill their prescriptions on their next scheduled visit, indicating a possible non-adherence problem.

The use of biologic DMARDs in rheumatoid arthritis pharmacotherapy presents added opportunities for community pharmacists to monitor and guide patients in a safe manner. Patients suffering from infections or recurrent infections are likely to seek the advice of the community pharmacists in relation to medications they can take. Patients on biologic DMARDs should therefore be reminded to interrupt their treatment with biologics until the infection is resolved. Vaccination is another aspect which features in community pharmacy setting. Community pharmacists should recommend the flu vaccine to all patients at high risk including patients on biologic DMARDs. Live vaccines, which may be acquired through community pharmacies, must not be administered to patients on biologic DMARDs. The community pharmacist will be able to identify such a contraindication and refer the patient accordingly.

These are a few examples of the contribution and role of the community pharmacists within a pharmaceutical care model for rheumatoid arthritis patients.

Community pharmacists are able to identify various pharmaceutical care issues and liaise with the hospital-based clinical pharmacist, thereby ensuring continuity of optimum individualised care within the primary care settings. Community pharmacists are able to identify patients who are not responding to the prescribed pharmacotherapy and whose quality of life is being severely impacted because of inefficacy.

5.3.1 Barriers to Community Pharmacy Pharmaceutical Care Models

Barriers to effectively resolving identified pharmaceutical care issues exist, despite the ability of the community pharmacists to identify such issues. This is because community pharmacists may not have easy access to the medication plan or discharge note outlined within the secondary care setting. They may not, at all times, have direct access to the patients' clinicians or the clinical pharmacists within the secondary care. Shared care guidelines and the use of health information technology such as the implementation of shared electronic patient records are examples of ways to overcome or decrease the communication barrier between the primary and secondary care setting [42–45]. Shared care guidelines are designed to assist healthcare professionals at different interface settings reach clinical decisions in a systematic approach thus allowing the seamless transfer of patients [46, 47]. A shared care model allows for improved co-ordination between secondary and primary care retaining the patients' well-being and quality of life at the centre of the service provision [48, 49].

Continuous education sessions organised with the aim of sharing with community pharmacists the latest evidence-based guidelines and recommendations on rheumatoid arthritis help to promote confidence of the community pharmacists in managing a complex condition such as rheumatoid arthritis and further improving the pharmaceutical care service offered to patients.

In order to achieve the best possible pharmaceutical care plan, pharmacists at both interfaces need to interact not only with each other and with clinicians but also with other healthcare professionals such as practice nurses, physiotherapists, occupational therapists and podiatrists who are involved in managing rheumatoid arthritis patients [50, 51].

Take-Home Messages
- Movement of patients across the care interface may result in medication problems.
- Pharmacists play an important role in medication reconciliation both on admission and on discharge.
- Hospital pharmacists are very often the last healthcare professionals whom patients discharged from the secondary care setting meet.

- Community pharmacists are often the first port of call to patients in the community setting.
- Through the implementation of pharmaceutical care models, community pharmacists can improve the quality of care of rheumatoid arthritis patients.
- Liaison between community pharmacists and hospital pharmacists working within the rheumatology field is essential to ensure optimum continuity of care.

Real Case Scenario 1
Mrs KC is a 45-year-old lady who has been suffering from rheumatoid arthritis for the past 15 years. She is currently on methotrexate 25 mg weekly and folic acid 10 mg weekly. Mrs KC has been recently seen by the rheumatologist who introduced etanercept 50 mg once weekly to her therapy plan. Mrs KC presents to the community pharmacy with a prescription for etanercept and admits to the community pharmacist that she is unsure as to how to take etanercept. The community pharmacist invites Mrs KC to a private area and shows the patient how to use the etanercept pen. The patient is encouraged to learn to self-administer etanercept. In order to ensure a good technique and boost the patient's confidence in using the pen, the pharmacist invites Mrs KC to visit the pharmacy to self-administer the next dose.

Real Case Scenario 2
Mr TR is a 65-year-old gentleman who presents to the pharmacy with a prescription to pick up his scheduled leflunomide 20 mg. As soon as he walks into the community pharmacy, the pharmacist notices that the patient is not his usual self. The pharmacist notices that the patient has swollen and tender joints in his hands. He admits that lately he has been suffering from early morning stiffness and he has pain mainly in his hands. The pharmacist urges the patient to visit his clinician as he might need treatment review and in the meantime dispenses an appropriate nonprescription analgesic.

Real Case Scenario 3
Mrs TR is a 78-year-old lady suffering from rheumatoid arthritis and diabetes mellitus. She has been admitted to the local hospital for management of congestive heart failure exacerbated by a community-acquired pneumonia. The pharmacist at the local hospital calls at the community pharmacy to confirm Mrs TR's treatment and ensure continuity of care since Mrs TR is a bit confused about her medications and it was difficult to develop an accurate medication history on admission.

References

1. Knight DA, Thompson D, Mathie E, Dickinson A (2013) Seamless care? Just a list would have helped! Older people and their carer's experience of support with medication on discharge home from hospital. Health Expect 16(3):277–291
2. Urban R, Paloumpi E, Rana N, Morgan J (2013) Communicating medication changes to the community pharmacy post-discharge: the good, the bad and the improvements. Int J Clin Pharm 35:813–820
3. Jones CD, Vu MB, O'Donnell CM, Anderson ME, Patel S, Wald HL et al (2015) A failure to communicate: a qualitative exploration of care co-ordination between hospitalists and primary care providers around hospitalised patients. J Gen Intern Med 30(4):417–424
4. American College of Clinical Pharmacy, Hume AL, Kirwin J, Bieber HL, Couchenour RL, Hall DL et al (2012) Improving care transitions: current practice and future opportunities for pharmacists. Ann Pharmacother 32(11):326–337
5. Hesselink G, Schoonhoven L, Barach P, Spijker A, Gademan P, Kalkman C et al (2012) Improving patient handovers from hospital to primary care: a systematic review. Ann Intern Med 157(6):417–428
6. Picton C, Wright H (2012) Keeping patients safe when they transfer between care providers: getting medicines right. Publisher: Royal Pharmaceutical Society 1–32
7. Fowells A (2013) Transfer of care can be risky business but it is in our interest to get it right. Pharm J 290:698
8. Johnson A, Guirgius E, Grace Y (2015) Preventing medication errors in transitions of care: a patient case approach. J Am Pharm Assoc 55(2):264–276
9. Duguid M (2012) The importance of medicine reconciliation for patients and practitioners. Aust Prescr 35:15–19
10. Duran-Garcia E, Fernandez-Llamazares CM, Calleja-Hernandez MA (2012) Medication reconciliation: passing phase or real need? Int J Clin Pharm 34(6):797–802
11. Ensing HT, Stuijt CCH, van den Bemt BJF, van Dooren AA, Karapinar-Carkit F, Koster ES et al (2015) Identifying the optimal role for pharmacists in care transitions: a systematic review. J Manag Care Spec Pharm 21(8):614–636
12. Kern KA, Kalus JS, Bush C, Chen D, Szandzik EG, Haque NZ (2014) Variations in pharmacy-based transition of care activities in the United States: a national survey. Am J Health Syst Pharm 71(8):648–656
13. Haynes KT, Oberne A, Cawthon C, Kripalani S (2012) Pharmacists's recommendations to improve care transitions. Ann Pharmacother 46(9):1152–1159
14. MeKonnen A, McLachlan A, Brien JE (2016) Effectiveness of pharmacist-led medication reconciliation programmes on clinical outcomes at hospital transitions: a systematic and meta-analysis review. BMJ Open 6:e010003. doi:10.1136/bmjopen-2015-010003
15. Unroe KT, Pfeiffenberger T, Riegelhaupt S, Jastrzermbski J, Lokhnygina Y, Colon-Emeric C (2010) Inpatient medication reconciliation at admission and discharge: a retrospective cohort study of age and other risk factors for medication discrepancies. Am J Geriatr Pharmacother 8(2):115–126
16. Beckett RD, Crank CW, Wehmeyer A (2012) Effectiveness and feasibility of pharmacist-led admission medication reconciliation for geriatric patients. J Pharm Pract 25(2):136–141
17. Buckley MS, Harinstein LM, Clark K, Smithburger PL, Eckhard DJ, Alexander E et al (2013) Impact of clinical pharmacy admission medication reconciliation program on medication errors in "high risk" patients. Ann Pharmacother 47:1599–1610
18. Galvin M, Jago-Byrne MC, Fitzsimons M, Grimes T (2013) Clinical pharmacist's contribution to medication reconciliation on admission to hospital in Ireland. Int J Clin Pharm 35(1):14–21
19. Lawrence DS, Masood N, Astles D, Fitzgerald CE, Bari AUI (2015) Impact of pharmacist-led medication reconciliation on admission using electronic medicines records on accuracy of discharge prescription. J Pharm Pract Res 45(2):166–173

20. Allende Bandres MA, Arenere Mendoza M, Gutierrez Nicolas F, Calleja-Hernandez MA, Ruiz La Iglesia F (2013) Pharmacist-led medication reconciliation to reduce discrepancies in transitions of care in Spain. Int J Clin Pharm 35(6):1083–1090
21. Geurts MM, van der Flier M, de Vries-Bots AM, Brink-van der Wal TI, de Gier JJ (2013) Medication reconciliation to solve discrepancies in discharge documents after discharge from the hospital. Int J Clin Pharm 35(4):600–607
22. Farley TM, Shelsky C, Powell S, Farris KB, Carter BL (2014) Effect of clinical pharmacist intervention on medication discrepancies following hospital discharge. Int J Clin Pharm 36(2):430–437
23. Bishop MA, Cohen BA, Billing LK, Thomas EV (2015) Reducing errors through discharge medication reconciliation by pharmacy services. Am J Health Syst Pharm 72(17):S120–S126
24. Caroff DA, Bittermann T, Leonard CE, Gibson GA, Myers JS (2015) A medical resident-pharmacist collaboration improves the rate of medication reconciliation verification at discharge. Jt Comm J Qual Patient Safety 41(10):457–461
25. Holland DM (2015) Interdisciplinary collaboration in the provision of a pharmacist-led discharge medication reconciliation service at an Irish teaching hospital. Int J Clin Pharm 37(2):310–319
26. Michaelsen MH, McCague P, Bradley CP, Sahm LJ (2015) Medication reconciliation at discharge from hospital: a systematic review of the quantitative literature. Pharmacy 3(2):53–71
27. Sebaaly J, Parsons LB, Pilch NA, Bullington W, Hayes GL, Easterling H (2015) Clinical and financial impact of pharmacist involvement in discharge medication reconciliation at an Academic Medical Centre: a prospective pilot study. Hosp Pharm 50(6):505–513
28. Karapinar-Carkit F, Borgsteede SD, Zoer J, Smith HJ, Egberts AC, van den Bemt PM (2009) Effect of medication reconciliation with and without patient counseling on the number of pharmaceutical interventions among patients discharged from the hospital. Ann Pharmacother 43(6):1001–1010
29. Phatak A, Prusi R, Ward B, Hansen LO, Williams WV, Vetter E et al (2016) Impact of pharmacist involvement in the transitional care of high-risk patients through medication reconciliation, medication education, and postdischarge call-backs (IPITCH Study). J Hosp Med 11(1):39–44
30. Johnson CM, Marcy TR, Harrison DL, Young RE, Stevens EL, Shadid J (2010) Medicine reconciliation in a community pharmacy setting. J Am Pharm Assoc 50:523–526
31. Sen S, Bowen JF, Ganetsky VS, Hadley D, Melody K, Otsuka S et al (2014) Pharmacists implementing transitions of care in inpatient, ambulatory and community practice settings. Pharm Pract 12(2):439
32. March G, Gilbert A, Roughead EE, Quentrell N (1999) Developing and evaluating a mode for pharmaceutical care in Australian community pharmacies. Int J Pharm Pract 7(4):220–229
33. Bernsten C, Bjorkman I, Caramona M, Crealey G, Frokjaer B, Grundberger E et al (2001) Improving the well-being of elderly patients via community pharmacy-based provision of pharmaceutical care. Drugs Aging 18(1):63–77
34. Farris KB, Fernandez-Llimos F, Benrimoj SI (2005) Pharmaceutical care in community pharmacies: practice and research from around the world. Ann Pharmacother 39:1539–1541
35. Christensen DB, Farris KB (2006) Pharmaceutical care in community pharmacies: practice and research in the US. Ann Pharmacother 40(7–8):1400–1406
36. Westerlund LT, Bjork HT (2006) Pharmaceutical care in community pharmacies: practice and research in Sweden. Ann Pharmacother 40(6):1162–1169
37. de Castro MS, Cassyano JC (2007) Pharmaceutical care in community pharmacies: practice and research in Brazil. Ann Pharmacother 41(9):1486–1493
38. George PP, Moliina JA, Cheah J, Chan SC, Lim BP (2010) The evolving role of the community pharmacist in chronic disease management – a literature review. Ann Acad Med Singapore 39(11):861–867
39. Mossialos E, Courtin E, Naci H, Benrimoj S, Bouvy M, Farris K et al (2015) From "retailers" to health care providers: transforming the role of community pharmacists in chronic disease management. Health Policy 119(5):628–639

40. Nazar H, Nazar Z, Portlock J, Todd A, Slight SP (2015) A systematic review of the role of community pharmacies in improving the transition from secondary to primary care. Br J Clin Pharmacol 80(5):936–948
41. Bayraktar A, Hudson S (2013) Design and evaluation of monitoring programme for methotrexate users in the arthritic population – a study at the primary and secondary interface. Turk J Pharm Sci 10(1):125–136
42. van Mil JWF, de Boer WO, Tromp THFJ (2001) European barriers to the implementation of pharmaceutical care. Int J Pharm Pract 9(3):163–168
43. Hardwick R, Pearson M, Byng R, Anderson R (2013) The effectiveness and cost-effectiveness of shared care: protocol for a realist review. Syst Rev 2:12
44. Hammond WE (2010) Seamless care: what is it; what is its value; what does it require; when might we get it? Stud Health Technol Inform 155:3–13
45. Rao S, Brammer C, McKethan A, Buntin MB (2012) Health information technology: transforming chronic disease management and care transitions. Prim Care 39(2):327–344
46. Hickman M, Drummond N, Grimshaw J (1994) A taxonomy for shared care for chronic disease. J Public Health 16(4):447–454
47. MacKay C, Veinot P, Badley EM (2008) Characteristics of evolving models of care for arthritis: a key informant study. BMC Health Serv Res 8:147
48. Madarnas Y, Joy AA, Verma S, Sehdev S, Lam W, Sideris L (2011) Models of care for early-stage breast cancer in Canada. Curr Oncol 18(Suppl 1):S10–S19
49. Lim A, Tan CS, Low BP, Lau CT, Tan TL, Goh LG et al (2015) Integrating rheumatology care in the community: can shared care work? Int J Integr Care 15:e031
50. Kristeller J (2014) Transition of care: pharmacist help needed. Hosp Pharm 49(3):215–216
51. Marion CE, Balfe LM (2011) Potential advantages of interprofessional care in rheumatoid arthritis. J Manag Care Pharm 17:S25–S29

Conclusion: Teaching Pharmaceutical Care of Rheumatoid Arthritis Patients to Student Practitioners: Imparting Care

"Knowledge is not understanding, understanding is not wisdom, wisdom is not empathy, empathy is not care. Care (however) adds quality." This is a quote by the late Professor Steve Hudson, who besides music, among other things in life, strongly held the pharmacy profession at heart. He passionately transmitted the very essence of pharmaceutical care concepts to his students both at an undergraduate and postgraduate level. The concept of imparting "care" not empathy toward patients in need of our service as pharmacists in order to continuously contribute to a higher level of quality of service provision was ingrained in each pharmacist coming in contact with him. This is exactly what pharmacy and pharmaceutical care is all about. Students can be thought to design and compile individualized care plans for their patients through various exercises, but the best practice is through direct contact with the patients themselves. It is through direct clinical experiences that we grow as pharmacists and in turn help our profession to further evolve along the years.

This book attempts to give an overview of the theory required to understand and gain wisdom into the rheumatoid arthritis as a condition. The authors of the book have where possible used clinical examples to illustrate pharmaceutical care issues encountered in rheumatoid arthritis patients. Yet, the best way to learn about rheumatoid arthritis and effectively care for the patients is through direct pharmacist-patient experience. Listening to the patients' concern is the best way for pharmacists to learn to care and subsequently effectively offer the best possible service.

Patient Experience

This is a brief first-hand overview of living with rheumatoid arthritis. I have been suffering and living with rheumatoid arthritis for the past 34 years. At the age of 18 years, I had the first symptoms of rheumatoid arthritis suffering from swelling and stiffness in my hands and knees. The pain in my knees hindered me from being able

© Springer Science+Business Media Singapore 2016
L. Grech, A. Lau (eds.), *Pharmaceutical Care Issues of Patients with Rheumatoid Arthritis*, DOI 10.1007/978-981-10-1421-5

to walk on my own, even for short distances. My parents immediately took me to our family doctor who referred me for further tests. The tests confirmed rheumatoid arthritis. Needless to say, I was deeply shocked and saddened to find myself diagnosed with rheumatoid arthritis, limited in movement and also in the activities of daily living. I was told it was a condition which is lifelong and that at that point in time, there was no cure. Before rheumatoid arthritis struck, I was a very active teenager living a normal life, wearing heels and enjoying partying and dancing. Rheumatoid arthritis limited all these joys and I found myself being helpless, needing help to walk around and do the basic things in life, let alone dancing and wearing heels!

Once confirmed rheumatoid arthritis, I started attending regular hospital visits. At the time I was prescribed soluble aspirin for the pain in addition to simple paracetamol. However this proved of little benefit and I had to learn to cope with rheumatoid arthritis. Soon after I was seen again in the hospital and was prescribed sulfasalazine to be taken three times daily. This seemed to work even though every now and then I would get an attack or flare up and I would require hospitalization for administration of intravenous methylprednisolone. Sometimes I would do away with the drip and get an intra-articular injection of steroid in the effected joint. As the condition progressed, I was prescribed gold injections which I took for 10 years. The condition continued to progress and when etanercept was launched, I was put on it in addition to methotrexate as a weekly dose. I learned to self-inject etanercept. Etanercept worked miracles and for the first time I felt I could live a "normal" life. However after a number of years, the condition hit back again and my specialist decided to switch me onto a different drug called infliximab. I have been on infliximab for at least 6 years now and so far the condition seems to have been suppressed. During my rheumatoid arthritis experience, I underwent a total elbow replacement procedure carried out in the United Kingdom. Living with rheumatoid arthritis is not easy. One has to learn to cope and adapt to living with the condition. It requires a lot of understanding and patience from our relatives and carers. However one cannot give up on life. Despite rheumatoid arthritis, I am married and have a son who is preparing to get married himself in the coming year and hopefully I will be able to slowly but surely aid in the wedding preparations. One way to overcome the condition is also by maintaining oneself educated as much as possible on the condition and the treatment provided. The healthcare team are after all always there to provide the necessary support so might as well maximize their service.

Patient Experience

I am a 44-year-old lady who was diagnosed at age 20. At the time I worked self-employed as a hairdresser and was dating my husband. At one point I started getting pain and swelling in my hands and wrists. My feet especially my knees and my ankles were swollen and painful. I did not give it much thought at first as I thought these were probably due to overdoing it at the hair salon. However as time went by, the symptoms remained and did not get better on weekends when I did not work. My future husband pushed me to visit the family doctor who ran a few tests and sent me off to the hospital for a visit at a rheumatology clinic. I was already a bit shaken having to go to a rheumatology unit without knowing what it entailed exactly. At the clinic, I was calmly and professionally told that I was diagnosed with rheumatoid arthritis. I was immediately started on methotrexate weekly tablets and prednisolone tablets among other medications. I was not very keen on starting the prednisolone since one of the symptoms was weight gain. The issue of methotrexate being teratogenic and that pregnancy was strictly forbidden while I was on methotrexate was discussed. At the time, having children was not planned. I could hardly take care of myself let alone plan to have children. My fiancé was very understanding and supportive. After approximately 4 weeks, I noticed a clear improvement in the symptoms. Eventually the condition was controlled even though I could not work long hours as a hairdresser as this tired me and I got occasional flare-ups if I overworked at work. Over the years, the condition progressed and I was administered various other drugs including etanercept and subsequently infliximab to successfully control the condition. I underwent total hip replacement at both hips and had to give up on my job as a hairdresser. The major disappointment in my life was the issue of not being able to try and have children. The issue was discussed several times with my specialist and my husband. The pros and cons were weighed each time and though my husband seemed to accept the fact that having children was not to be in our case, and at times for my benefit was not in favor of a decision to have children, I, myself, found it a bit more difficult to accept. Nonetheless, looking back on life today at 44 years, I believe I have the determination to go on and smile to the world. I am an aunt to a beautiful nephew and have a loving family, an adorable husband, and a great team of specialists at the hospital and in the community pharmacy who go out of their way to help me.

Glossary

ACER Average cost-effectiveness ratio
ACR American College of Rheumatology
ADR Adverse drug reaction
AIMS Arthritis Impact Measurement Scales
ANA Antinuclear antibody
BOOP Bronchiolitis obliterans organizing pneumonia
BSR British Society for Rheumatology
BHPR British Health Professionals in Rheumatology
CBA Cost-benefit analysis
CBC Complete blood count
CCA Cost-consequence analysis
CEA Cost-effectiveness analysis
CCP Cyclic citrullinated peptide
CI Confidence interval
CMA Cost-minimization analysis
CRP C-reactive protein
CUA Cost-utility analysis
DAS Disease activity score
DHFR Dihydrofolate reductase
DMARDs Disease-modifying antirheumatic drugs
bDMARDs Biologic disease-modifying antirheumatic drugs
boDMARDs Biosimilar disease-modifying antirheumatic drugs
sDMARDs Synthetic disease-modifying antirheumatic drugs
DNA Deoxyribonucleic acid
E. coli *Escherichia coli*
ECG Electrocardiogram
ECHO Economic, Clinical, Humanistic Outcomes
ESR Erythrocyte sedimentation rate

EULAR European League Against Rheumatism
FH4 Tetrahydrofolate
FSI Functional Status Index
HAQ Health Assessment Questionnaire
HIV Human Immunodeficiency Virus
HLA Human leukocyte antigen
HRQOL Health-related quality of life
ICER Incremental cost-effectiveness ratio
ID Insufficient date with respect to RhMAT criterion
IL-1 Interleukin 1
IL-6 Interleukin 6
LDL Low-density lipoprotein
LGY Life years gained
MACTAR McMaster Toronto Arthritis Patient Preference Disability Questionnaire
MAT Medication Assessment Tool
MCP Metacarpophalangeal
MCH Mean corpuscular hemoglobin
MCHC Mean corpuscular hemoglobin concentration
MCV Mean corpuscular volume
MTP Metatarsophalangeal
NICE National Institute for Health and Care Excellence
NHP Nottingham Health Profile
No^J Justified nonadherence to RhMAT criterion
No$_{UJ}$ Unjustified nonadherence to RhMAT criterion
NSAIDs Nonsteroidal anti-inflammatory drugs
NNTH Number needed to harm
NNTT Number needed to treat
PPI Proton pump inhibitor
QALY Quality-adjusted life years
QWB Quality of Well-Being Index
RA Rheumatoid arthritis
RF Rheumatoid factor
RhMAT Rheumatoid Arthritis Medication Assessment Tool
RNA Ribonucleic acid
SF36 Medical Outcomes Study Short Form-36
SIP Sickness Impact Profile
TFCQ Toronto Functional Capacity Questionnaire
TNF Tumor necrosis factor
UDHR Universal Declaration of Human Rights
VEGF Vascular endothelial growth factor

Index

A
Abatacept, 29, 31
Absolute risk, 45–46
Acute phase reactant, 9, 10
Adalimumab, 20, 28, 31, 47, 48, 57
Adherence, 55, 59–61, 64–65, 73
Adherence rate, 61
Aetiology, 4–5
Alcohol, 24
American College of Rheumatology, 8, 21, 22,
    30, 60
Amyloidosis, 6
Anaemia, 7, 9, 25
Anakinra, 20, 28, 29, 31, 59
Analgesics, 21–23, 61
Anti-cyclic citrullinated peptide (anti-CCP),
    9–11, 13
Anti-nuclear antibody (ANA), 7, 9
Aspirin, 20, 21
Autoimmune disease, 3, 11
Azathioprine, 27, 31, 58

B
Biologic drugs, 22, 29–31
Breastfeeding, 10, 31, 62
British Society for Rheumatology, 30, 31, 56, 60

C
Caplan's syndrome, 6
Cardiovascular disease, 7, 11, 47
Carpal tunnel syndrome, 6
CD20, 21, 29
Certolizumab, 20, 28, 31
Ciclosporin, 27, 31, 58

Clinical pharmacist, 53, 59, 74
Community pharmacist, 40, 51, 72–75
Co-morbidities, 5, 7, 11, 21, 47
Complete blood count (CBC), 9, 58, 59, 62
Compression syndromes, 6
Congestive heart failure, 29, 75
Corticosteroids (steroids), 21
Cost, 30, 39, 41–47
Cost-benefit, 43–45
Cost-consequence, 43
Cost-effectiveness, 43–44, 47, 48
Cost-minimisation, 43
Cost-utility, 43, 45
Counselling, 58, 60, 65, 72, 73
C-reactive protein (CRP), 9
Cytokines, 4, 7, 21, 26, 28
Cytomegalovirus, 4

D
Deformity, 4, 5
Diagnosis, 8–12, 21, 61
Direct costs, 42, 47
Disease activity score (DAS28), 47
Disease modifying anti-rheumatic drugs, 33,
    34, 37, 66
Disease progression, 4, 11, 20, 21, 23, 54, 65
Drug therapy problems, 54–57, 73
Dry mouth, 6

E
Episcleritis, 6
Epstein–Barr virus, 4
Erythrocyte sedimentation rate (ESR), 9, 10,
    30, 62

© Springer Science+Business Media Singapore 2016
L. Grech, A. Lau (eds.), *Pharmaceutical Care Issues of Patients
with Rheumatoid Arthritis*, DOI 10.1007/978-981-10-1421-5

Etanercept, 20, 28, 29, 31, 47, 48, 58, 75
European League Against Rheumatology
    (EULAR), 7, 8, 10, 22, 30, 31, 60,
    62
Extra-articular manifestations, 4–6, 11

F
Felty's syndrome, 7
Functional disability, 63
Fusion protein, 28, 29

G
Genetic factors, 4
Glomerulonephritis, 6
Golimumab, 20, 28, 31
Guidelines, 21–24, 30, 31, 56, 59, 60, 64, 65,
    74

H
Health, 39–45, 47, 51, 60, 63–65
Health assessment questionnaire (HAQ), 48,
    49, 63, 64
Health related quality of life tools, 63–65
Hepatitis B, 29, 58, 59, 62
Hepatitis C, 29, 59, 62
Hepatomegaly, 7
Hospital pharmacist, 72
Human Immunodeficiency Virus (HIV), 29
Hydroxychloroquine, 22, 26–27, 30, 31, 57,
    58, 61

I
Immunodeficiency, 24, 26
Incremental costs, 42
Indirect costs, 42
Inflammatory arthritis, 1, 5
Infliximab, 20, 28, 29, 31, 47, 48, 57, 59
Intangible costs, 42
Interleukin, 4, 7, 20, 21, 26, 28, 29

J
Joints, 1–3, 5, 8–11, 21, 75
Juvenile idiopathic arthritis, 1

L
Leflunomide, 10, 20–22, 26, 30, 31, 43, 57,
    58, 61, 75
Liver disease, 12, 24

Liver impairment, 24, 27, 56
Lymphadenopathy, 7

M
Magnetic resonance images (MRI), 8
Malignancy, 7, 30, 62
Manifestations, 4–7, 11
Medication adherence, 55, 64–65, 73
Medication assessment tool, 60, 65
Medication reconciliation, 72, 74
Metacarpophalangeal joints, 10
Metatarsophalangeal (MTP) joints, 8, 10
Methotrexate, 4, 10, 20–25, 28–31, 48, 57–59,
    61, 62, 64, 73, 75
Monitoring, 21, 30, 43, 55–60, 62
Monoclonal antibody, 28, 29
Mononeuritis multiplex, 7
Monotherapy, 22, 23, 28–31, 48
Morbidity, 6, 7, 42, 45
Morning stiffness, 5, 54, 75
Mycoplasma, 4

N
Neurological manifestations, 6
Neuropathy, 6, 27
Neutropenia, 7, 59
Non-steroidal anti-inflammatory drugs, 21, 22
Number needed to treat (NNTT), 46, 47

O
Obliterative bronchiolitis, 46–48
Onset, 3–5, 8, 10, 22
Opportunity costs, 42
Osteoporosis, 7, 54, 57
Outcomes, 21, 41–44, 51, 54, 63

P
Pharmaceutical care, 53–65, 72–74
Pharmaceutical care issues, 53–65, 73, 74
Pharmaceutical care plan, 54, 72–74
Pharmacist, 40, 43, 51, 53–55, 57–65, 72–75
Pharmacoeconomics, 39–51
Pharmacotherapy, 8, 19–31, 51, 54, 55, 60,
    62–65, 72–74
Pharmacy, 39, 41, 53, 55, 71, 73–75
Pregnancy, 10, 11, 31, 62
Prevalence, 3
Prognosis, 4, 9, 11–12, 21
Psoriatic arthritis, 1, 48
Pulmonary fibrosis, 6, 25

Pulmonary manifestations, 6
Pyramidal approach, 20–22

Q
Quality-adjusted life-years (QALYs), 45, 47, 48
Quality of life, 2, 5, 11–12, 21, 39, 42, 49, 51, 54, 55, 60, 62–65, 74

R
Relative risk, 45–46
Renal impairment, 24, 26, 27, 56
Rheumatoid arthritis, 1–12, 19–31, 39–51, 53–65, 71, 73–75
Rheumatoid factor (RF), 7, 9
Rheumatoid nodules, 5
RhMAT, 54, 60–62, 65
Rituximab, 20, 29–31

S
Scleritis, 6
Scleromalacia, 6
Serology, 8
Side-effects, 25, 29, 30
Sjogren's syndrome, 6
Skin, 5–7, 27
Smoking, 4
Sodium aurothiomalate, 20, 27, 30, 61
Splenomegaly, 7
Spondyloarthropathies, 1, 5
Squeeze test, 8

Subluxation, 6
Sulfasalazine, 20–22, 25, 30
Symptoms, 5, 6, 8, 10, 11, 21, 54, 73
Synovial membrane, 3–5

T
Teratogenic, 31
Thrombocytopenia, 7
Tocilizumab, 20, 29, 31, 57, 59
Toxicity, 20, 25, 27, 30, 42
Transitional care, 71–75
Tuberculosis, 28, 58, 59
Tumour necrosis factor (TNF), 4, 20, 21, 26, 28–31
Tumour necrosis factor inhibitor, 4

U
Ulceration, 6, 24, 25
Ultrasound, 8

V
Vaccination (vaccines), 73
Vasculitis, 6, 7

W
Washout procedure, 26

X
X-ray, 4, 8, 12, 58, 62